WHO PLAYS?,
WHO PAYS?,
WHO CARES?:

A Case Study in Applied Sociology,
Political Economy and the
Community Mental Health Centers Movement

SYLVIA KENIG

Political Economy of Health Care Series
Series Editor: Ray Elling

Baywood Publishing Company, Inc.
AMITYVILLE, NEW YORK

Library of Congress Catalog Number: 91-36243
ISBN: 0-89503-092-6 (Paper)
ISBN: 0-89503-093-4 (Cloth)

Library of Congress Cataloging-in-Publication Data

Kenig, Sylvia.
    Who plays? who pays? who cares? : a case study in applied
sociology, political economy, and the community mental health
centers movement / Sylvia Kenig.
        p.   cm. — (Political economy of health care series)
    Includes index.
    ISBN 0-89503-093-4 (cloth). — ISBN 0-89503-092-6 (paper)
    1. Community mental health services—Economic aspects—United
States.   2. Community mental health services—Political aspects-
-United States.   3. Social psychiatry—United States.   I. Title.
II. Series.
    RA790.6.K46   1992
    362.2'2—dc20   91-36243
                                                                         CIP

Copyright Releases

Copyright permission has been obtained from the following:

This work is dedicated to my parents,
Esther Leibovitz Kenig and
Isadore Joel Kenig

Acknowledgments

The author wishes to express thanks to Dr. Ray H. Elling, editor of the Baywood Publishing Company series on the Political Economy of Health. Dr. Elling has steadfastly served as an inspiring teacher and a dedicated scholar/activist.

Thanks also go to the members of Baywood Publishing Co., especially to Mr. Norman Cohen and to Mr. Stuart Cohen, without whose help this book would not have been possible.

Work on this manuscript was supported through financial aid from the University of Connecticut Health Center and from the University of South Carolina–Coastal Carolina College. The latter was especially generous in its support of the research and writing necessary for this volume. Thanks go to USC–Coastal Chancellor, Dr. Ronald G. Eaglin and to Dean Betsy Puskar of the College of Natural and Applied Sciences for their help and support. Thanks also go to the Coastal Department of Sociology and its Chair, Dr. Joan Piroch. In addition, the Department of Sociology of USC–Spartanburg was kind enough to offer office space during work on the manuscript. Special thanks to Ms. Bonnie Senser for her work on the draft copy.

For their scholarly insights and unfailing friendship during the initial research, the author thanks Helen Raisz, Lois Haignere, Catherine McDonald, Chris Witzel, Carol Goodenough, and Ellen Gruenbaum. For his guidance and help during the middle phase of this project, thanks go to Dr. Spurgeon Cole and Dr. John Ryan.

To my husband and children I owe a special debt for their love and understanding—Ken Smith, Amanda Smith, and Eric Smith.

Contents

List of Tables

CHAPTER 1

Introduction

This is a book of many parts. In a sense it is a study of a social movement—the community mental health centers (CMHC) movement. In another sense it is an analysis of the political economy of that movement and of the applied sociological literature developed within that movement. The over arching intent of the book is to demonstrate through one case study, that the applications of the intellectual products of social scientists are influenced by the political economic context in which those products are applied.

In this first chapter the logic of the analysis is set forth. The reader is introduced to the building blocks of the analysis including: 1) an idea of the central concept of "community"; 2) a brief discussion of applied sociology; and 3) a discussion of the sociology of knowledge with special emphasis on the sociology of applied knowledge. The chapter ends with a brief look at the logic of the analysis as presented in each succeeding chapter.

COMMUNITY

The concept of community is certainly one of the most frequently discussed terms in the social and behavioral literature. At first glance it might call up images of comfortable houses surrounded by well-tended lawns and children playing ball in the local park. Or it might call up harsher images of decaying houses jammed with low income families.

Students of sociology might be more highly sensitized than most persons to the many possible meanings of community. They might think of the works of Tonnies, Durkheim, or contemporary sociologists of community such as Roland Warren, who in 1973, warned against an overly romanticized view of the community and "the equally remote conception of a territorially undifferentiated mass society . . ." [1, p. 408]. A sociologically oriented reader might even be moved to ask: Is there such an entity as "community" in modern America? Perhaps the consciousness of living in a certain neighborhood is the most that modern Americans can experience of "community." Undoubtedly many of the functions which were thought to be part of community in the past have been removed from local geographic localities. The legal system, the schools, the medical care corporate complex, and the political system have all taken over some of what formally might have been thought of as community functions.

The concept of community has been addressed by sociologists in the United States at least since the flourishing of the discipline in the midyears of the century. As the patterns of urban, suburban, and rural life changed, so too did the concept.

The many approaches to the concept of community have been summarized probably in at least as many forms as there are texts on the topic itself. One typical example is the typology offered by Hassinger and Pinkerton in 1986 in their introductory text on community, *The Human Community*. The authors divide schools of community into: The ecological approach—community as space; the ethnographic approach—descriptions of actual communities usually developed through participant observation; and the organizational approach including variations on the themes of closed systems, groups in conflict, or open systems. The authors, own definition covers considerable ground—community for them is "an area in which groups and individuals interact as they carry on daily activities and in which regularized means of solving common problems have been developed" [2, p. 35].

Clearly community has been a dynamic concept as well as a dynamic entity. Authors have repeatedly dealt not only with the thorny problem of defining the entity but describing the processes which catalyzed groupings of persons into a "community." Theories of community development addressed this perplexing issue. Hunter in 1978 suggested that community development could be conceptualized in a series of stages from that of residual neighborhood—a feeling of physical proximity to neighbors, to emergent communities which exhibited a sense of shared sentiments, to conscious communities which developed an acknowledged internal structure, to the final stage of vicarious or symbolic communities where persons who do not actively participate in the community still maintain a sense of connectedness to it [3].

Indeed the search for the ultimate meaning of community occupied the imaginations of scholars, of social activists, and of utopian dreamers looking for perfection of the human person through perfection of the human collectivity.

Precisely because community is such a common and ambiguous term, it is a useful marker for tracing the implicit assumptions of authors who employ it. In other words, it offers many opportunities to ask: What did the author imply about the larger society by using the concept of "community" in the way he/she did? This is the question addressed in this book. The core of the analysis presented here can be summed up by asking why the term community was used in the way it was during distinct political economic phases of the community mental health movement. The fact that the term was used in non-sociological works makes this a study in applied sociology, and it is meant to be an analysis useful to all those who work in sociological practice and the behavioral sciences.

APPLIED SOCIOLOGY

According to Elizabeth Clarke, in her 1986 summary of sociological practice which was written for members of the Sociological Practice Association, the term applied sociology was used frequently at the turn of the century [4]. From the very beginning of the discipline, some sociologists used their special skills in theory production and methodology to attack "real world" problems for purposes other than scholarly publication. And from the beginning there has been a debate over the discipline boundaries surrounding applied work. Questions were often asked about whether the products of such work were truly sociological? Were they perhaps more appropriately classified as social work? Were they a type of social psychology or social psychiatry?

The debate continues today both within what has been traditionally called academic sociology and within the ranks of those who label themselves as applied sociologists. Sociologists who train for and work within such settings as mental health centers, nursing homes, or programs for drug and alcohol abuse often call themselves clinical sociologists. The Sociological Practice Association certifies those who undertake a certifying examination to be CCSs, Certified Clinical

Sociologists. Whether formally certified or not, clinical sociologists are found working with individual clients, groups, or entire "communities."

Sociologists who specialize in activities such as evaluating social welfare or health programs, or who are employed in a variety of policy-oriented consulting firms are more apt to label themselves applied sociologists. One of the newer terms used as an umbrella concept to capture this multiplicity of roles is sociological practice.

In this book, applied sociology refers to social concepts, models, and theory which are used in written material to address real world situations. For the most part, the applications are not by sociologists but by other professionals working within the general field of mental illness treatment. Although many different professions and occupations were represented in the CMHC movement, the literature addressed here is chiefly from the fields of community psychiatry and community psychology. These two were chosen as central to the CMHC movement and broadly representative of the types of applied social theory seen in the movement's literature.

The sociological schools of thought analyzed are consensus and conflict theory. The content of these schools of theory is captured by focusing on the use of the concept "community" in one specific literature, the literature of the community mental health centers (CMHC) movement.

As the title of this book suggests, the major assertion of the analysis is that sociological theory is applied in these other disciplines in ways that reflect the needs of the larger political economic context. Unlike what some philosophers of knowledge have argued [5] it is not the contention here that scientific (or in this case, social scientific) knowledge grows and changes in response to the rather autonomous intellectual activity of scientists. Rather, it is argued that the products of intellectuals are significantly limited and shaped by the economic and political atmosphere within which their works are created [6]. The fact that, in this study, the works are sociological and are published for non-sociologists, makes the relationship between the products and their context all the more interesting and useful for persons working in applied fields.

THE SOCIOLOGY OF KNOWLEDGE

Sociologists of knowledge are concerned with the development of systems of thought in relationship to the material and cultural context of that thought. The Modern Dictionary of Sociology, defines the sociology of knowledge as "the aspect of sociology that is concerned with the relationship between knowledge or systems of thought (scientific, religious, philosophical, aesthetic, political, legal, etc.) and social and cultural factors" [7, p. 406].

One of the major factors which differentiates one sociologists of knowledge from another is the emphasis placed on the importance of the political economic context in intellectual production. The following pages present a sense of this debate.

MARX

A significant portion of our contemporary sociology of knowledge can be traced back to basic assertions made by Marx. As Marx wrote in his German Philosophy, "Life is not determined by consciousness, but consciousness by life" [8, p. 75]. In the same work, he argued, "The ideas of the ruling class are, in every age, the ruling ideas: i.e., the class which is the dominant 'material' force in society is at the same time its dominant 'intellectual' force. The class which has the means of production at its disposal, has control at the same time over the means of mental production, so that in consequence the idea of those who lack the means of mental production are, in general, subject to it" [8, p. 78]. Such assertions were the product of a relatively young Marx, and were later dismissed by some critics as lacking in the sophistication of the more mature Marx. Nonetheless, the words carried a power and conviction that influenced both Marx's contemporaries and a later school of theory called "humanist Marxism." (See Chapter 2 for further discussion of this school of theory.)

MANNHEIM

Following on Marx, Mannheim was profoundly interested in the relationship between systems of thought and their socio-political contexts [9-11]. According to Mannheim, an analysis of intellectual production did not depend on analysis of individual motives, or even on the analysis of the truth contained within the system of thought. For Mannheim, general or partial systems of thought were always value laden, ideological, and systematically linked to the concrete situations in which they were produced. The sociology of knowledge, therefore, was built by systematically exploring these links.

One of the most important ideas developed by Mannheim was that of the social generation [9-11]. He wrote that humans who experienced the same historical conditions and reacted to them in similar ways, shared a consciousness, a system of thought. In this way, Mannheim elaborated on Marx's earlier writings which posited a strong connection between material reality and human consciousness.

Mannheim believed that intellectuals acted as members of any of a number of different classes or parties. Despite this, he also believed that intellectuals could escape the concrete situations of classes and move beyond them through their intellectual products. The potential of this rather special ability was the essence of the creativity of intellectuals, the ability to transcend the hold of historical situations.

One of the most persistent criticisms of Mannheim was that he reduced all thought to mere products of specific historical periods, products without intrinsic validity of their own—a charge that could be leveled equally at the early Marx. This criticism of relativism also called into question the ability of intellectuals to understand their own products since they were caught in the trap of their own historical situations. This criticism continues to challenge today's sociologists of knowledge, but as will be shown later in this chapter, some contemporary theorists have posited a type of "willing one's self" out of the hold of class.

GRAMSCI

Antonio Gramsci's life story reads as a tragic tale indeed. In addition to suffering from physical deformity all his life, he ended his years slowly dying in prison. Despite his hardships, Gramsci, especially in his Prison Notebooks [12], brilliantly articulated a theory of the centrality of culture, systems of belief, in class struggle.

Gramsci explored the process of ideological development in its relationship to the material conditions of the times. According to him, these conditions and life experiences formed the filters through which classes understood themselves through art, history, and through all knowledge. Gramsci argued that when such understandings were gradually unified into systems of thought, they became ideologies, organic ideologies as he called them because of their relationship to life.

As a unified system of thought was able to find expression throughout culture, it gained ideological dominance, i.e., cultural hegemony. But unification and dominance were also related to the dominance of the elite class which used this cultural hegemony to support its own position and to turn nondominant classes against one another.

The struggle for class liberation, Gramsci argued, had to develop along cultural lines as well as through material or economic changes. An alternative, unified, organic ideology had to be articulated from the life experiences of the working class in order for its members to break the hold of cultural control by the elites. The leaders in this cultural struggle were the intellectuals.

For Gramsci, the emergence of ideologies was neither automatic nor uniform. Culture did not emerge directly from change in the material conditions of life, nor did it spring fully developed from the pens of intellectuals. It was created in bits and pieces, slowly, as the processes of life unfolded. Many such pieces co-existed at any one historical moment, and dominance was only achieved gradually as the system of thought grew.

Gramsci's analysis carried the sociology of knowledge beyond Mannheim's work in several respects. Gramsci's emphasis on the continuous creation and struggle of organic ideologies in any one historical period improved upon the more static concept put forth by Mannheim.

As Gramsci wrote [12, p. 407]:

> The claim, presented as an essential postulate of historical materialism, that every fluctuation of politics and ideology can be presented and expounded as an immediate expression of the structure, must be contested in theory as primitive infantilism, and combated in practice with the authentic testimony of Marx, the author of concrete political and historical works.

Gramsci clearly saw the subtle but omnipresent struggles between class-based systems of thought and material reality. The give and take between life experience and consciousness, and the relationship between this unfolding process and class struggle are fully recognized in his writings, as is the active role of the intellectual.

CONTEMPORARY AMERICAN SOCIOLOGY OF KNOWLEDGE

In the politically charged atmosphere of the 1960s, many American sociologists began to turn renewed attention to the sociology of knowledge. As political ideologies turned colleague against colleague and student against professor, it seemed necessary for scholars to explain to themselves exacting how their intellectual products related to the turmoil encroaching on their universities. In 1967, for example, Howard Becker, a well known sociologist of deviance, wrote an article asking: "Whose Side Are We On?" [13]. In it he voiced the concern that sociology provoked charges of bias by refusing to give credence and deference to an established status order. Becker's way out of the bind of whether to side with subordinates or superordinates was to make clear the limits of one's study, marking the boundaries beyond which research finding could not be applied.

A somewhat angry response came from a then rising star of sociology, Alvin Gouldner, in his 1968 article, "Sociologist as Partisan: Sociology and the Welfare State" [14]. Gouldner charged that emotional blandness, implied by Becker, was not an effective antidote for partisanship. Instead, doing the sociology of underdogs often meant doing it sympathetically but from a white, middle-class perspective. Gouldner's answer was to work toward a sociology for human unity rather than an "empty-headed" partisanship. Two years later, Gouldner was to publish a more fully developed work on the same general theme.

GOULDNER

In 1970 two landmarks in contemporary American sociology of knowledge were published, Gouldner's *The Coming Crisis of Western Sociology* [15], and Friedrichs' *A Sociology of Sociology* [16].

The Coming Crisis of Western Sociology made a convincing case that the slide of American sociology away from the classic historical debate between functionalism and Marxism (see Chapter 2), was importantly related to the changing role of sociologists in American society. As with earlier sociologies of knowledge, the theme was the importance of the relationship of intellectual production to its material and sociopolitical context. As Gouldner reaffirmed [15, p. 47]:

> Rooted in a limited personal reality, resonating some sentiments but not others, and embedded in certain domain assumptions, every social theory facilitates the pursuit of some but not of all courses of 'action' and thus encourages us to change or to accept the world as it is, to say yea or nay to it. In a way, every theory is a discreet obituary or celebration for some social system.

But Gouldner's social system analysis was not that of Mannheim or Gramsci. Rather than developing an analysis of class struggle as the foundation for his sociology of knowledge, Gouldner more broadly labelled conservative functionalism as the dominant theory in academic sociology of the United States; Marxism as the dominant theory within Soviet sociology. The convergence of these into a conservative administrative sociology produced sociology "whose aim is to protect and strengthen the existent master institutions of . . . society, rather than to examine them as a source of society's problems" [15, p. 475].

Gouldner echoed the hopes of other sociologists of knowledge in predicting that a revitalized sociological theory could be a tool of progressive social change. He believed that a liberated theory could be authored by liberated sociologists. The key was to produce what Gouldner termed a reflexive sociology. This self-critical and self-aware work was to be "based upon an awareness that the academician and university are not simply put upon by the larger world, but are themselves acting and willing agents in the dehumanizing of this larger world" [15, p. 512].

FRIEDRICHS

A fascinating contrasting work by Friedrichs, *A Sociology of Sociology,* also was published in 1970. Friedrichs traced the dominance of the priest over the prophet in contemporary American sociology. He also called upon sociologists to engage in a new dialogue among schools of thought, arriving at a new self-awareness of themselves and their works. But unlike Gouldner's active conceptualization of sociologists as change agents, Friedrichs conceived of a more mild "witnessing" process. Sociologists in this scheme would witness the profound religious and philosophical debates between priests and prophets.[1]

A SOCIOLOGY OF APPLIED SOCIOLOGICAL THEORY

In all these works, the primary focus was on scholarly production within the university (although Gouldner did include in his attack administrative sociology in the service of the welfare state). Certainly these sociologists of knowledge agreed that intellectual products were not created as free-floating systems of thought, but that each served as an ideology which supported or undercut classes or interests in the specific historical situation. Academic theorists were seen as acting to

---

[1] The works cited here in no way reflect the entire field of contemporary sociology of knowledge. They are meant only to provide two distinct vantage points from which to view the field.

legitimate or to criticize, or in rare moments, to transcend their own material conditions.

The question now must be asked: What about the application of sociological theory outside of the discipline itself? Are the same constraints at work? Are other forces evident?

One type of answer was given in a work published in 1986, *Professional Powers: A Study of the Institutionalization of Formal Knowledge* by Elliot Freidson [17]. Although not concerned specifically with the application of sociological knowledge, Freidson traced major currents in the development of knowledge by tracing the rise and fall of professions, their structural positions, and their technologies. As with earlier works, he included special attention to issues of medicine. Freidson stressed the rather special constraints on the application of knowledge by professionals who worked outside of the traditional academic settings, and he looked at social controls on the growth of professions, their market positions, and legal sanctions. In many ways this analysis parallels the current work. The major difference comes in Freidson's placing of the history of impressions at the core of the analysis and using the political economy as a sort of secondary limiting factor. In the current analysis, the political economy is placed at the corner, and the intellectual products of varying professionals are seen as largely responding to market and State needs. This difference will become clearer as the analysis unfolds.

Still another type of answer to the questions posed regarding the production of applied knowledge was given almost a decade earlier in the much quoted, Sociology for Whom?, authored by Alfred McClung Lee in 1978 [18]. After analyzing the value-laden bases of sociological work, and the sanctions brought to bear against sociologists who dared to dispute conventional methods, Lee argued that sociology could be liberated in the sense of making it more humane. Lee compared what he conceptualized as humanist sociology to the dominant American approach. Humanist sociology, he argued should, among other things, be people centered, ethical, dedicated to an acceptance of social change, a product of carefully trained scientists who value intimate observation and creative intellectual ferment [18, p. 94]. As to the process of building such a sociology, Lee suggested that humanist scholars should work in a "society of cooperative friends"; that they should be critical of the abuses of power and privilege in their ranks; and that they should explore and publicize the manipulative strategies and propaganda to which so much of the media, politics, religious apologists, and formal education are devoted [18, pp. 221-223]. Although Lee had a critical vision of the realities of intellectual production, he also voiced an optimism about its possibilities, especially when carried out in concert with like-minded individuals. His vision gave rise to the Association for Humanist Sociology which included members from a broad range of social and behavioral sciences.

LESSONS FROM THE PROFESSION OF HISTORY

Of course sociologists have not been the only scholars to ask such questions concerning the products of their labors. Professional historians in the United States, for example, have also been much concerned with questions of how and why the content of their academic products change over time and under differing conditions.

A fascinating look at the type of debates in which these scholars participate can be found condensed in a series of articles published in 1989 by *The Journal of American History* [19]. The topic of this particular issue was how and why radical history became a legitimate subfield within the discipline during the 1960s and 1970s when before it frequently had been scorned or ignored.

The lead article in this issue of *The Journal* was "Radical Historians and the Crisis in American History," by Jonathan Wiener [20]. In it the author described how the consensual model of history dominated the American profession in the 1950s and was supported in this domination by intimidation of radical historians during the McCarthy era. At length, radical historians were able to overcome this domination because central figures within their ranks were able to establish themselves in supportive academic environments, were able to attract interested students, were able to find outlets for their scholarship in journals of radical history, and were able to draw "intellectual energy" from events in the larger society.

The antiwar movement of the 1960s, along with the civil rights movement, and later the women's movement, provided the backdrop against which questions of class struggles, capitalist domination, and revolutionary change became acceptable topics for mainstream scholarly history journals. The convening of the Socialist Scholars Conferences in the mid 1960s allowed these academics to engage in dialogues with a broad range of interested students and activists. The activists themselves also founded radical journals and distributed radical scholarship in the form of pamphlets such as those sponsored by the Students for A Democratic Society (SDS).

But the tone and content of radical historical scholarship changed significantly as the 1960s drew to a close. The assassinations of Dr. Martin Luther King and Robert Kennedy, and the rioting in Chicago during the Democratic Convention vividly reflected a transformation of anger from rhetoric to reality by radicals on both ends of the political spectrum. SDS disintegrated, radical fought radical, and the senior New Leftists who were now legitimated within academe began to soften their language as they achieved tenure within their departments.[2]

As addressed through argument and rebuttal in this issue of *The Journal,* and in society at large [21], authors continued to argue over just how much radicals had lost in their new legitimated status. Christopher Lasch [22] wrote in *The Journal* that the works of radical historians had become every bit as predictable and tedious as any academic product, and Carl Degler [23] argued in response to John Higham [24] that radical scholarship had not been rejected because of its ideology but because the evidence presented was judged to be inadequate.

THE PRODUCTION OF SCHOLARSHIP, ITS CONTEXT AND APPLICATION

All of this may be summed up as by Alfred McClung Lee in asking: Sociology (or history) For Whom? But this seems to capture only one bit of the larger picture. It's not only Scholarship for Whom?—although that does bring the consumer into the production process, it's also scholarship by whom and for what purpose? Phrased here the question is expanded to: Who Pays? Who Plays? and Who Cares?

These questions form the basis of understanding how the application of bits of social theory, in this case the concept of community, are integrated into scholarly discourse in any particular political economic period.

REFERENCES

1. R. L. Warren, *The Community in America,* (3rd Edition), Rand McNally, Chicago, 1973.

[2] This issue is now being hotly debated in the media and on campuses. Conservatives are charging that leftists from the 1960s and 1970s are instituting a new type of censorship in the form of "political correctness."

2. E. Hassinger and J. R. Pinkerton, *The Human Community*, Macmillan Publishing, New York, 1986.
3. A. Hunter, Persistence of Local Sentiments in Mass Society, in *Handbook of Contemporary Urban Life*, D. Street et al., (eds.), Jossey-Bass, San Francisco, 1978.
4. E. J. Clarke, *Sociological Practice: Defining the Field*, Sociological Practice Association, New York, 1986.
5. T. S. Kuhn, *The Structure of Scientific Revolutions*, University of Chicago Press, Chicago, 1962.
6. S. Kenig, The Use of Theory in Applied Sociology: The Case of Community Mental Health, *The American Sociologist, 18*:3, pp. 242-257, 1987.
7. G. A. Theodorson and A. G. Theodorson, *Modern Dictionary of Sociology*, Thomas Y. Crowell Company, New York, p. 406, 1969.
8. K. Marx, *German Ideology*, translated by T. B. Bottomore in *Karl Marx, Selected Writings in Sociology and Social Philosophy*, McGraw Hill Book Company, New York, 1956.
9. K. Mannheim, *Essays on the Sociology of Knowledge*, Routledge and Kegan Paul, Inc., London, 1952.
10. K. Mannheim, *Essays on the Sociology of Culture*, Routledge and Kegan Paul, Inc., London, 1956.
11. K. Mannheim, *Ideology and Utopia*, Routledge and Kegan Paul, Inc., London, 1960.
12. A. Gramsci, *Selections from The Prison Notebooks*, International Publishers, New York, 1971.
13. H. Becker, Whose Side Are We On?, *Social Problems, 14*, pp. 239-247, Winter, 1967.
14. A. W. Gouldner, The Sociologist as Partisan: Sociology and the Welfare State, *The American Sociologist*, pp. 103-116, 1968.
15. A. W. Gouldner, *The Coming Crisis of Western Sociology*, Basic Books, New York, 1970.
16. R. W. Friedrichs, *A Sociology of Sociology*, The Free Press, New York, 1970.
17. E. Freidson, *Professional Powers: A Study of the Institutionalization of Formal Knowledge*, University of Chicago Press, Chicago, 1986.
18. A. McClung Lee, *Sociology for Whom?*, Oxford Press, New York, 1978.
19. D. Thelen, A Round Table: What Has Changed and Not Changed in American Historical Practice?, *The Journal of American History, 76*:2, pp. 393-486, 1989.
20. J. Wiener, Radical Historians and the Crisis in American History, 1959-1980, *The Journal of American History, 76*:2, pp. 399-434, 1989.
21. R. Kimball, *Tenured Radicals: How Politics Has Corrupted Our Higher Education*, Harper & Row, New York, 1990.
22. C. Lasch, Consensus: An Academic Question?, *The Journal of American History, 76*:2, pp. 457-459, 1989.

23. C. N. Degler, What Crisis, Jon?, *The Journal of American History*, 76:2, pp. 467-470, 1989.
24. J. Higham, Changing Paradigms: The Collapse of Consensus History, *The Journal of American History*, 76:2, pp. 460-466, 1989.

CHAPTER 2

Models of
Applied Social Theory

APPLIED CONSENSUS THEORY

What were the priestly and prophetic sociologies described by Friedrichs [1] and the western functionalism and Marxism described by Gouldner [2] which so thoroughly influenced American sociology? Why were they seen as ideological opposites? And what were the conceptual tools each theory offered to behavioral scientists who applied social theory in their own work? In this chapter, the traditions of consensualism and conflict theory will be explored, especially those elements relevant to applied sociology and to the community mental health centers movement in particular. It should be noted again that various names such as consensualism, functionalism, and structural functionalism refer to what here is drawn together into one idealized model of the same tradition of social theory. Likewise, prophetic sociology and Marxism are here drawn with a broad brush under the image of conflict theory. Although purists may object to this because there are differences within schools of theory, for purposes of this analysis consensualism is conceptualized as one school and conflict theory as the other major tradition against which it has competed in the minds and in the literature of American sociology in this century.

In a sense, consensual sociologists are like jigsaw puzzle enthusiasts. They see their task as studying both the contours of the total puzzle and the fit of each specific piece into the whole. Depending on the school of consensualism, attention may be focused on the total puzzle and its larger pieces, or it may be focused on the individual pieces and how, in everyday life, persons try to bend or stretch the pieces to fit the spaces available. The consensualism of Talcott Parsons is an example of the first kind of approach; the consensualism of Robert Merton is an example of the second approach. The similarities among such consensualists are primarily based on their assumptions that society functions as a rather static, closed system. They adopt for their writings the dispassionate scientific language of the times in which they wrote. Professionals from other disciplines such as the lawyers or physicians often readily adopted both the assumptions and the language of consensualism because it tended to legitimate their professional domains and it offered a language easily understood by non-sociological professionals. Unlike the passionate dialectical talk of the prophetic conflict theorists, the calm and reasoned tone of consensus social theory appeared accessible and reassuring to non-sociologists. Alfred McClung Lee [3], a longtime critic of consensualism, turned his critical eye toward the social system approach when he wrote [3, p. 21]:

> A 'social system' is only a patchwork of many devoutly held myths. It is seen differently, and those myths are interpreted differently, in each of society's groups. Whether the 'system' can legitimize something—can give a sense of security and stability by sanctioning one's status, influence, or career—depends upon what is happening to a particular myth in that patchwork.

When the myth supported the assumed expertise of mental health professionals, as it did in much of the mental illness literature, it was easily molded to legitimate their practice.

Consensualists also acted as the priests described by Friedrichs [1] when they brought to their writings assumptions as to the correct or proper functioning of each unit of the social system. Norms, values, roles were defined as if mid-century, white, middle-class America was the ultimate normative standard against which all other value systems should be judged. When consensualists turned their attention beyond the borders of the United States or across decades and centuries, they tended to slip rather naturally into evolutionary models of social change [2, 4]. As late as 1967, Talcott Parsons, in his *Sociological Theory and Modern Society* [5], continued to emphasize the conditions for social stability as including adaptation, goal attainment, integration, and pattern maintenance—the conceptual building blocks which he had developed to fit his earlier social systems scheme. All tended to support a very static view of the puzzle pieces mentioned earlier. His attempt to address issues of social change in his final work, *The Systems of Modern Society* [6], resulted in his explication of four major evolutionary universals represented by the legal system, membership and citizenship, the market system, and bureaucratic organization. According to Parsons, voluntary change formalized distinctions among these four processes of structural change: the economic process of adaptive upgrading, the political process of structural differentiation, the integrative process of inclusion of new units, and the latent pattern maintaining processes of value generalizations. In simple terms these processes referred to how the puzzle pieces might have to be shaved a bit around the edges to make them fit as the total puzzle contours change slightly over time.

If sociologists had trouble interpreting such language, it is understandable that non-sociologists found it challenging. But on the positive side, when applied to the work of other occupational groups, such concepts proved to be supportive of professional domains partially through its very mystification of professional language. It is also easy to understand the attraction such concepts held for lawyers, economists, and politicians whose activities were implicitly assumed to be central and necessary to the processes of social stability and of social change.

Many critics have grappled with Parson's undoubted influence on American sociology. Perhaps the most eloquent, C. W. Mills [7], charged him with fuzzy language and simplistic thinking, among other problems. Turner [8] charged that Parsonian structural functionalism was needlessly repetitious and circular in its reasoning—mirroring a similar critique by Dahrendorf [9] who likened Parsonian society to a utopia, an ahistorical entity built on universal value consensus with an overriding emphasis on stability.

Other authors sought to excuse Parsonian consensualism from this criticism by arguing that his theory was, after all, not a fully developed theoretical system but was an ideal typical representation of society [10]. Parsons himself wrote in 1961 that his theory, ". . . is not yet a logico-deductive system but rather a temporal and historical series of contributions toward the development of such a system" [11, p. 321]. And certainly Parsons' work was a significant reason why American sociological at mid-century had gained the respectability within academe that it had. It presented to the public a way to think about society which seemed scientific and supportive of basic middle-class ideology.

Still basic problems remained for theorists. Lockwood, in his oft cited essay, "Some Remarks on the Social System" [12], summarized much of the critique which had been voiced by mid-century by stressing the conclusion that the Parsonian emphasis on order and stability made change and disorder appear abnormal and pathological. According to Lockwood, in reality, scarce resources and forced choices about the distribution of those resources made societal tension inevitable. Conflicts were always structured into the very fabric of society—something Parsonian consensualism was never fully able to integrate into the social system model.

Merton, another important consensualist, addressed this issue of nonconformity, non-consensual behavior, in relationship to the social system [13]. Merton's famous paradigm of cultural goals and individual adaptations offered an easily understood typology for classifying everyone from autistics to vagabonds. Merton defined conformity as the acceptance of both goals and means; innovative as the acceptance of goals but rejection of means; ritualism as the rejection of goals but the acceptance of means; retreatism as the rejection of both goals and means; and rebellion as the rejection of goals and means with the substitution of new goals and means in place of the old ones. This simple but powerful approach offered a way to think of nonconformity as structured into the system. The integrity of the basic social system model could thus be maintained while addressing dysfunctional aspects of it.

Another of Merton's major contributions was his application of what was called middle range theory. He discussed community, for example, in terms of information sharing. In his essay, "Patterns of Influence: Local and Cosmopolitan Influentials," [13, pp. 387-420], Merton defined community not in terms of the abstract and somewhat fleshless concepts offered previously by Parsons, but in terms of communication patterns as they linked people together in a systematic yet dynamic interactional network.

Despite attempts by Merton and others to breathe new life into consensualism, its implicit background assumptions remained in tact, especially the assumption that behavior should be defined as "normal" only if it fit the assumed societal consensus and pathological if it did not. This point was made forcefully by Horowitz who stressed the consensual assumption that consensus in every situation is assumed to be functionally relevant [14]. Horowitz argued that within the consensual tradition, Parsons and Merton equated rebellion with alienation and conformity with equilibrium, thereby ruling out the possibility that a condition of rebellion is consonant with equilibrium or that extreme cases of consensus may create social or personal disequilibrium. Horowitz's analysis made use of the timely example of the Freedom Riders, protesters in the 1960s civil rights struggle. These persons who defied the local norms that black people were supposed to sit only at the back of public buses, purposely rode buses sitting in the front seats. Such non-normative behavior might easily be considered by the traditional consensualists as pathological.

In what stands as probably the most closely reasoned critique of Merton's consensualism, the philosopher Ernest Nagel [15], made the case that in order to establish that observed behavior is fulfilling the functions which Merton implied, an author would have to describe fully the underlying structure of the society and the exact function of each part for the whole. Alternatives could then be said to be either supporting or undercutting these necessary and sufficient functional conditions. Without such a complete analysis, Nagle argued, variations from any one arrangement could not be termed to be either functional or dysfunctional for the immediately perceived societal organization.

In referring back to the jigsaw puzzle metaphor, the major criticisms of consensualism could be stated in terms of the attempt by the puzzle doer to deal with pieces which clearly did not fit the puzzle. Something might be wrong with the total puzzle, maybe pieces from several different puzzles had been thrown together in one batch and those that didn't fit were deviant, i.e., belonged to another puzzle. Or it might be, as some theorists began to suggest about society, that perhaps the picture itself was changing all the time and as soon as one piece was placed, its fit might or might not compliment that of its dynamic neighbor.

This dynamic approach to society was more easily addressed by the conflict sociological tradition.

APPLIED CONFLICT THEORY[1]

In place of the social systems model constructed by Parsonians or the middle range theory of Merton, conflict theorists elaborated on the philosophical tradition of historical materialism. This meant focusing

[1] It should be noted that the forms of conflict theory discussed in this work are generally variations on the themes set down by Karl Marx. However, since the variations are legion, marxism is spelled with a small "m" in order to differentiate the general school of theory from the actual work of Marx.

on the mode of production, such as capitalism, at a given historical moment. The contradictions inherent in each mode, such as those related to class struggle, were central to the analysis. The causal model rather than being evolutionary was dialectical, again focusing on the contradictions within society at any given point in history. This theoretical tradition was term Marxism by Gouldner [2] and prophetic sociology by Friedrichs [1]. It posited quite different background assumptions and carried quite different ideological implications from the consensual approach.

As represented in Table 1, these differences included both the conceptual units of the theory and its model of societal change.

Unlike the consensual view of society in which individuals were conceptualized as being socialized to the prevailing value system in order to promote stability, conflict theory assumed that conflict and struggle were at the heart of the capitalist societal process. In the conflict view, individuals were socialized to the particular values, norms and roles of their own class. The appearance of social stability was maintained as a fiction for the purposes of supporting the dominant class or interest groups within that class, i.e., class factions.

For consensual authors, attention was most easily directed toward what was perceived as "real" and "normal" for white, middle-class members of society. According to conflict authors, it was conflict which both held society together and potentially pulled it apart. Conflict theorists within the United States often felt a close kinship to their European forebears, retaining, as they had, an intense interest in and awareness of historical political economic struggle on this worldwide scale. It was within this tradition that such conflict theorists as Andrew Gunder Frank [16] traced the growth of capitalist colonialism and the underdevelopment in the Third World. Such sweeping analyses differed not only in scope from the more modest tasks addressed by many American consensualists but also in their basic conceptual frameworks. The historical dialectical materialism of conflict analysis ran counter to the rather static orientation of the consensualists which often ignored historical changes. This meant, as will be explored in later chapters, that those behavioral scientists who adopted conflict theory were rather naturally drawn toward allying themselves with powerless groups, were active on behalf of social change efforts, and their writings were marked by a tone of righteous indignation regarding perceived societal injustices.

Some social theorists who are called conflict theorists do not fit the model outlined here. They base their approaches on non-class value

Table 1. Comparison of Basic Elements of Conflict
and Consensus Sociology

	Consensus	Conflict
Unit of Analysis	System Subsystem Community	Norms,World System Nation Class
What Holds Society Together?	Social systems exist in a state of dynamic equilibrium and tend toward self-maintenance.	Society exists as a contra-diction-ridden, growing and changing compromise between classes or class factions.
	Society consists of highly integrated and mutually interdependent subsystems.	Classes or factions exist in opposition to one another and are defined within specific historical periods. They are defined with reference to the group's relations to the means of production.
	The basis of system inte-gration is value consensus. Issues of authority are often presented in terms of assumed value con-sensus; formal social control agents such as the police and army are assumed to represent enforcement of this.	The basis of social process is struggle over power. Authority is conceptualized only in relation to each class; agents of social control enforce the needs of the dominant class.
	Norms, values, roles are consensually agreed upon and support structure and function.	Norms, values, roles are related to each class. Nonconformism may emerge from stuggle against class-base norms.

Table 1. (Cont'd.)

	Consensus	Conflict
	The division of labor is built upon patterns of needs and it reflects natural system differentiation in structure and function.	The division of labor must be understood as relating to each class at one point in history.
What pulls society apart or what causes society to change?	Change is conceptualized within a framework of evolution. History engenders change through a variety of internal and external sources causing subsystem differentiation.	Change is conceptualized within a framework of historical materialism: sources of change are defined through the contradiction between and within classes.
	Change creates mutually reciprocal exchanges and adjustments among subsystems which tend to return the system to equilibrium and to minimize structural change. When this is not possible, the system may collapse and be replaced by a new one.	In periods of quiescence, change is minimized through the hold of the dominant class by overt and covert social control (force and ideology) and by maintenance of the existing political economic formation. When class conflict reaches peak periods, control is weakened or broken.

conflict or on other conflicts not directly tied to materialist class analysis. One example is the work by Rapoport on mathematical modeling of conflict. This fascinating approach, set forth for example, in Rapoport and Chammah [17] presents a view of interpersonal conflict in which oppositional parties interact in a zero-sum game. The questions asked by the authors refer to the conditions under which one might predict the various behaviors given the probabilities of action. Although this indeed addresses social psychological conflict, it is not grounded in the neo-marxian tradition, and it does not assume the inherent social injustices and their historical causes implicit in the prophetic tradition. It also does not carry the ideological overtones which the traditional prophetic approaches carry. For this reason, only those works which do fit this tradition are here termed conflict theory.

To return to the puzzle metaphor, it can be said that while Parsons, Merton and other consensualists labored long and hard to construct their jigsaw puzzle approach to society, conflict analysts were laboring equally vigorously to convince their audience that neither puzzle frame nor pieces were adequate representations of social process, a process which was too fluid to be represented by such concepts. To conflict theorists, frame and pieces kept moving and shifting their configuration under the influence of historical class struggle, a struggle which intensified or weakened depending on the specific historical conditions.

Rather than the concept of social system which was found so frequently in the consensual literature, conflict theorists focused on the concept of class. Social system implied a "system" which might have boundaries which were either rather rigid or rather permeable. Nonetheless, such boundaries enclosed what was thought of as a distinct entity, one with a series of subsystems which displayed some degree of interdependence and integration. In the later, more sophisticated models of ecosystems (as will be discussed in Chapter 7), even these subsystems were conceptualized as dynamic, giving way to a succession of human societal forms. Nonetheless, change was still thought of as taking place within the given system, or within the given ecological nitch, as the social ecologists might term it. This basic concept of system was antithetical to the dialectical approach of the conflict theorists because it implied that a population was organized around consensual norms, values, roles in a rather rigid division of labor. Where and how the boundaries of the system were drawn mattered less than the fact that drawing such boundaries was an exercise in idealism. Defining class, for the conflict theorists was an exercise in historical materialism, i.e., it had a real world referent in a given historical period.

Saying this does not mean that conflict theorists could agree on what that real world definition of class ought to be. Despite the fact that class was the basic building block of concept theory, it remained problematical both to theorists and to social activists. Class remained such a slippery issue for conflict theorists partially because its definition depended on differing historical modes of production, and because conflict theorists differed as to the centrality of economic relations, political relations, and/or social relations in the definition of class. Even within the writings of Marx himself can be found a significant shift from an early concern with social forces of production and consciousness to a later concentration on economic relations, especially as displayed in his last work, *Capital*.

This is not to say that Marx's writings were contradictory. Marx stressed the social aspect of economic formations even in his late work. He reflected this nowhere more clearly than in his contention that human labor formed the basis of value in the productive process. His distinction between production for use by the populace and production for profit, especially under capitalism, led to the conclusion that under capitalism, workers were often occupied with the production of useless but profitable goods and services. Accordingly, capitalism was largely dependent on creating commodity fetishism—the need to own useless material symbols of wealth. The surplus created under capitalism needed outlets not found in truly productive labor and so the sociopolitical formation tended increasingly to create such nonproductive goods as military hardware [18]. This process and others related to the fundamental conditions of capitalism were what conflict theorists saw as pathological, rather than the non-compliance with norms highlighted by the more microanalytical approach of American consensualists.

Conflict theorists discussed socialization but they didn't emphasize conformity to middle-class norms, values and roles. Instead, they wrote of consciousness and alienation which were central topics of what became known as humanists marxism, a branch of neo-marxism based importantly on the early writing of Marx and on later developments, especially in the Frankfurt School of theory. Many marxists believed that the perception of reality was filtered through categories of class-based social experience. In this manner, the very acts of knowing or perceiving were dialectical and political. For such analysts, the basic question of knowing, was not whether the supposed consensually agreed upon view of society was the correct one, but who was served by the dominant view of society.

Much of this work on consciousness, which became central to later applied writings on social psychiatry, was produced in Frankfurt Institute for Social Research. The Institute was founded in 1932 in Frankfurt, Germany. Leading figures in the Institute included Adorno, Marcuse, and Fromm, all of whom fled Nazism and brought their work to the United States at mid-century. This tradition continues to profoundly influence the application of conflict social theory, especially in the behavioral sciences.

A prime example of this analysis is found in the writings of Herbert Marcuse [19] who struggled to unite the insights of Marx with those of

Freud. Marcuse introduced two new terms of the literature of social psychiatry; surplus repression and the performance principle. The first referred to Freud's belief that civilization emerged from psychological repression. Marcuse elaborated on this idea by suggesting differing levels of exploitative social arrangements led to differing levels of "surplus repression" above the baseline repression needed for minimal social order. In other words, people who were caught in exploitative capitalist socio-economic systems, experienced the unconscious need to repress a tremendous amount of psychological injury which they daily experienced. A certain amount of such repression, especially repression of sexuality and other biological needs, was necessary for social order. But capitalism produced surpluses of this repression. According to marcuse [20, p. 16]:

> In the advanced capitalist countries, the radicalization of the working classes is counteracted by a socially engineered arrest of consciousness, and by the development and satisfaction of needs which perpetuate the servitude of the exploited.

The performance principle extended Freud's analysis of the pleasure principle. Pleasure seeking behavior, according to this view, was in conflict with the reality principle or goal-oriented behavior. In goal-oriented behavior, the ego was primarily concerned with the performance principle and surplus repression. People had to carry out goal-oriented behaviors in order to exist in society. Expressions of sexuality, which were so obvious and accessible in modern society, were not reflections of liberated genital sex according to Marcuse. They were expressions of "desublimated sexuality." a sexuality which supported and served the repressive productive process within capitalism. Humans became commodities, as was sex, to be bought and sold through alienated relationship in the economic marketplace. False needs were developed and perpetuated by profit seeking individuals, and perverted the striving for true sexual liberation as well as for economic liberation [20, p. 91].

Marcuse's work, in many respects, reflected the general direction of theory development within humanist marxism and the Frankfurt School. This approach, although firmly based in humanistic concerns of exploitation and alienation, did not carry the same class-based, revolutionary message as did the more hard line, orthodox marxism. Differences within schools of conflict theory also emerged in approaches to science. The Frankfurt School rejected standard forms of empiricism as reifying—making seem as real—exploitative social forms. According to this critique, what most scientists uncritically accepted as standardized operationalism and measurement were really just one approach among many to understanding reality. The approaches they adopted were usually static rather than appropriately dynamic and inclusive of contradictions. To counteract this reification, conflict theorists attacked science as the attempt to separate subject from object. According, for example, to Therborn, writing about the Frankfurt School, "Immutable scientific laws of society were the expression of a world in which human relations had become things beyond human control and the separation of different scientific disciplines revealed a specialization which destroyed the totality and historicity of human experience" [21, p. 65]. According to orthodox marxists, objectivity was the hallmark of the mature Marx. In focusing on economic relations, according to the orthodox authors, Marx had freed himself and his theory from earlier liberal tendencies which muddled conceptualization with too much emphasis on societal and psychological processes.

The major thrust of criticism directed toward consensualism focused on its lack of ability to deal with history and change, and its conservative bias. The major criticism directed toward conflict theory dealt with its lack of precise conceptualizations and its identification by others as revolutionary, communistic, un-American, or simply too apt to support anti-establishment social activism.

Typical criticisms leveled by social theorists were that conflict theory was built on imprecise conceptualizations and a fuzzy casual model [8]. Conflict theorists were often seen as polemicists rather than as constructive social theorists. The fact that they often allied themselves with social change movements supported this charge. Many conflict theorists gladly acknowledged their polemical bent, propounding the view that theory grew out of social action in the form of praxis—the joining of theory and action. As Gouldner wrote, the full impact of conflict theory on American sociology is an unwritten history because mainstream American functionalism [2, p. 448]:

> . . . developed in a middle-class society where Marxism was politically anathema, where the taint of Marxism could cripple academic careers, where Marxism was often dismissed out of hand as an outdated theory or as a mere ideology or as a 'religion' by those same people who otherwise professed a respect for religion.

Such warnings carried special import for those concerned with applying theory beyond the confines of academe.

The two major schools of theory discussed here, conflict and consensus theory, were not alone in the pages of social theory textbooks and the labels applied to them varied. They are adopted here because of their opposing ideological implications and because of their long history of dominance in sociology. For these reasons, they provide a useful framework for the present analysis.

Other approaches to theory abound in sociological texts. One of the most recent and most exciting is presented by Spector and Kitsuse in their 1987 work, *Constructing Social Problems* [22]. These authors focus particular attention on developing a logically unified approach to what become defined as "problems" for American society. They break what here is termed priestly sociology into a number of different schools of theory including functional etiology, normative sociology, and value conflict sociology. The first is identified with such concepts as dysfunction or social disorganization. The second uses such language as norms and value consensus. The third, value conflict theorists are seen as placing more emphasis on objective conditions but often implicitly accepting the disorganization/dysfunction approach. Unfortunately Spector and Kitsuse do not include marxism and neo-marxism as a category of theory for analysis in their work. Their value conflict school does not rest on class-based analysis but is built on a rather free-floating interest group view.

Despite the absence of the prophetic school from their analysis, the authors do document how approaches to social problems shift as arenas of discourse change, as roles of the sociologists change, and as audiences for their work change. Many fascinating cases from psychiatric literature are discussed as their argument proceeds. They trace the story of how homosexuality was re-conceptualized within the psychiatric diagnostic scheme from a disorder to an acceptable choice of sexual orientation [22, pp. 19-20].

In another fascinating case study, Spector and Kitsuse follow the complex tale of how, in the 1970s, American psychiatric and legal professionals began a long struggle over investigating claims by a Soviet dissident biologist of political misuses of psychiatry in the Soviet Union. Canadian and American psychiatric organizations began investigations, and it was hoped that action would be taken at the upcoming World Congress of Psychiatry in 1970. Meanwhile, a judge who had been part of the First United States Mission on Mental Health to the USSR a year earlier, David L. Bazelon, was drawn into the controversy by being asked to examine more closely the interface between the law and psychiatry in the USSR. Judge Bazelon argued that political misuse of psychiatry was not confined to the USSR. The American Psychiatric Association agreed to study this issue, but the choice of study participants soon became a major issue in itself, along with choice of research methodology and data. These concerns soon became central, overshadowing concern in the initial issue. The APA Committee appointed to study the case was angrily disbanded. After the judge was severely criticized by many prominent figures in American psychiatry for his role in this clash, he was ultimately granted an award by the psychiatrists for distinguished service to his work on behalf of psychiatry. As Spector and Kitsuse point out, this case highlights the importance of understanding the definition of "the problem" within the dynamic political context in which it is defined and analyzed.

Drawing on this case study and their overall critique of past approaches, the authors present their own way of understanding social problems. While not willing to suggest that all social problems follow a similar natural history, they do suggest that a logically consistent analytical method includes four stages which can be summarized as follows: 1) a group identifies and defines some condition as offensive or harmful; 2) officials recognize the legitimacy of this group and respond; 3) the original claims re-emerge with criticism of the official response; and 4) alternative responses are created [22, p. 142]. The strength of this approach is its recognition of the fluidity and variety of reactions to "problems" and their connection to the political context. Still, this analysis stopped short of conceptually tying the rise of oppositional interest groups to specific sectors of the political economy such as O'Connor's monopoly, competitive, and state sectors. Such a microanalytical framework could have anchored the seemingly independent rise and fall of interests in an over arching historical process. Spector and Kitsuse might have analyzed the case as a struggle between the interests of the State and of the monopoly sector psychiatric professionals. In the end, as one might have predicted, the interprofessional rivalries were muted and unity on behalf of State interests was ultimately upheld.

An interesting sidelight on this issue comes in the research of Wagenfeld and Robin [23] in 1976 when they explored the question of whether CMHC professionals extended their roles into other professional arenas such as education or the law. Those authors found that CMHC professionals did not "boundary bust," for the most part. They kept within their own turfs as the above model suggests.

Nonetheless, Spector and Kitsuse did recognize the importance of the professional contexts in which problem definitions arise and their impact on theory. They wrote [23, pp. 66-67]:

> When the resources for which various disciplines compete are scarce, theories may be advanced to lay exclusive claim to specific areas of research or to maintain control of the existing organization of academic specialization . . .
>
> Just as departments may attempt to gain exclusive control in conflicts with other disciplines, they may also form alliances within the university for the same purpose . . .
>
> . . . Just as subject studied by sociologists seldom view themselves as they are viewed by researchers, it is not surprising that sociologists do not subject their own activities to detached observation and analysis. However, their statements about causation of social phenomena, their attitudes toward interdisciplinary research, and their defense of the logic of the organization of disciplines within the university cannot be understood as a reflection of an empirical reality external to and independent of statements made about them.

In the present study of applied theory, theories are shown to be reflections of professional domains, such as those highlighted by Spector and Kitsuse, and of a more far reaching process of the balance between dominant and non-dominant ideologies within the larger political economy. The following chapter builds on this assertion by briefly tracing the rise of several dominant psychiatric theories and their implicit sociological assumptions.

REFERENCES

1. R. W. Friedrichs, *A Sociology of Sociology*, The Free Press, New York, 1970.
2. A. W. Gouldner, *The Coming Crisis of Western Sociology*, Basic Book, New York, 1970.
3. A. McClung Lee, *Sociology for Whom?*, Oxford Press, New York, 1978.
4. J. Toby, Parson's Theory of Social Evolution, *Contemporary Sociology, 1*:5, pp. 395-401, 1972.
5. T. Parsons, *Sociological Theory and Modern Society*, The Free Press, New York, pp. 204-205, 1967.
6. T. Parsons, *The Systems of Modern Society*, The Free Press, New York, 1971.
7. C. W. Mills, Grand Theory, in *The Sociological Imagination*, C. W. Mills (ed.), Oxford Press, New York, 1959.

8. J. Turner, *The Structure of Sociological Theory*, The Dorsey Press, Homewood, Illinois, 1974.
9. R. Dahrendorf, Out of Utopia, *American Journal of Sociology, 73*, pp. 115-127, 1968.
10. T. Abel, *The Foundations of Sociological Theory*, Random House, New York, 1970.
11. N. J. Demerath, III and R. Peterson (eds.), *System Change and Conflict*, The Free Press, New York, p. 321, 1967.
12. D. Lockwood, Some Remarks on the 'Social System,' *British Journal of Sociology, 7*, pp. 134-146, 1956.
13. R. Merton, *Social Theory and Social Structure*, The Free Press of Glencoe, 1957.
14. I. L. Horowitz, Consensus, Conflict and Co-operation: A Sociological Inventory, *Social Forces, 41*, pp. 177-188, 1962.
15. E. Nagel, A Formalization of Functionalism with Special Reference to Its Application in the Social Sciences, in *System Change and Conflict*, N. J. Demerath, III and R. Peterson (eds.), The Free Press, New York, pp. 77-94, 1967.
16. A. G. Frank, *Dependent Accumulation and Underdevelopment*, Monthly Review Press, New York, 1979.
17. A. Rapport and A. M. Chammah, *Prisoner's Dilemma: A Study in Conflict and Cooperation*, University of Michigan Press, Ann Arbor, 1965.
18. P. A. Baron and P. M. Sweezy, *Monopoly Capital*, Monthly Review Press, New York, 1966.
19. H. Marcuse, *One Dimensional Man*, Beacon Press, Boston, 1964.
20. H. Marcuse, *An Essay on Liberation*, Beacon Press, Boston, 1969.
21. G. Therborn, The Frankfurt School, *New Left Review, 63*, 1970.
22. M. Spector and J. I. Kitsuse, *Constructing Social Problems*, Aldine de Gruyter, New York, 1987.
23. M. O. Wagenfeld and Stanley S. Robin, Boundary Busting in the Role of the Community Mental Health Worker, *Journal of Health and Social Behavior, 17*, pp. 112-122, 1976.

CHAPTER 3

Social Psychiatry in Historical Perspective: an Uneasy Combination of Models of Mind and Models of Society

In the preceding chapter, two major schools of sociological theory were introduced along with the assertion that these theories implied opposing assumptions as to society's process and change. In this chapter, the application of these theories will be explored in their historical context, particularly as they influenced the development of American social psychiatry. Such analysis can be generalized to any of a number of disciplines which combine models of mind and of society. The major theme here will be that although the model of society may be adopted in rather an *ad hoc* fashion, it nonetheless implies certain background assumptions which reflect specific implicit ideological orientations. These hidden ideological assumptions then profoundly limit and direct the applied literature in which they are used.

FROM MORAL TREATMENT TO THE FREUDING OF AMERICA: 1700-1940

From the very birth of the United States in the 1700s, theories of madness were developing out of an uneasy synthesis between

European models of mind and society. The nascent American "profession" of psychiatry was organizing its domain around both a biological and social view of insanity. The biological, along with a genetic and somatic orientation were to come to dominate the literature of the profession. Social models eventually receded to the background.

Dr. Benjamin Rush, known as the father of American psychiatry, covered a wide range of behaviors in his categorization of insanity. In addition to detailed analysis of what today might be termed alcoholism, he diagnosed opposition to the American revolution as the mental illness "revolutiona" [1, p. 49].

Moral treatment, the core approach adopted in early American psychiatry, was based on a view of the human mind as extremely impressionable. As Ruth Caplan wrote in here extensive history of community psychiatry in nineteenth century America [2, p. 301]:

> The essence of moral treatment was the belief that, because of this great malleability of the brain surface, because of its susceptibility to environmental stimuli, pathological conditions could be erased or modified by corrective experience.

This belief lent an optimistic tone to early attempts at treatment; cure was not only possible but was likely under the correct social circumstances.

Moral treatment was recommended for ailments ranging from mania to melancholia. A host of causative factors were identified including [3, p. 46]:

> predisposition existed by novel reading; ill health caused by severe fanaticism; frustrated enterprise; perplexity in his pursuit; and repelled eruption . . . one hospital reported tight lacing as a causative factor in insanity.

Since much of the blame for distress was laid to social causes, treatments often consisted of placing patients in what were conceptualized as supportive social surroundings. These surroundings were modeled on the norms of those in control of the treatments and, for example, for women they often included forced resocialization into the restrictive gender roles of the day [4]. An interesting example of this comes from the history of one of the earliest and most prestigious asylums of the day, The Hartford Retreat. Its first two patients were a man and a woman. The male was described in the institution's records as "a male, single, thirty-six, suffering from the result of 'fanaticism', and a young woman, twenty-six, who had broken down recently from overtaxing the intellect with difficult studies" [3, p. 19].

Asylum building and the medicalization of mental distress found a great supporter in the person of Dorothea Lynds Dix, an activist who crusaded in the mid 1800s for hospital reform and federal support for care. Dix, along with a somewhat later but similar crusader, Clifford Beers, himself hospitalized on several occasions for mental illness, brought issues of mental treatments to the national consciousness. Beers founded an organization which was to become the National Association for Mental Health, a powerful interest group which backed the expanded availability of treatment sites. It was through such efforts that psychiatry organized as a sphere of interest in the private sector.

The 20th century brought with it a shift in psychiatric interest from moral treatment to Social Darwinism. The shift changed the theoretical emphasis from somatic treatments and environmental support to belief in the biological roots of insanity. A new and rather pessimistic tone now pervaded the literature. Again, according to Ruth Caplan [2, p. 301]:

> The insane were seen as an alien influence, creatures of another kind, now classed once more with other species of degenerates'; criminals, paupers, deaf mutes, retarded and so on. All groups were to be treated in the same way, by isolation and sterilization.

The dominant psychiatric approach to mental illness turned away from manipulating the social environment to controlling the genetic makeup of the individual. The eugenics movement was spread nationwide as discussion groups formed to discuss every new idea related to selected breeding.

The shift toward individualistic and somatic treatments was fueled in the United States as asylums, formerly seen as placid retreats for troubled minds, were being filled with waves of immigrants. The Irish famine and economic depressions in many European nations fueled massive worldwide migration. Immigrants to the United States were often viewed not only as objects as disgust, but, as the *American Journal of Insanity* described them, as carriers of "the germs of weakness, poverty and disease" [2, p. 294]. Asylums became the repositories for these displaced masses.

The gulf between social and somatic theories of mental illness was addressed by several theorists in the 20th century, both by those practicing in the United States and also medical missionaries in other lands. Adolf Meyer was one of the foremost influences on psychiatry during this decade. Meyer insisted that social relationships within the family and the community were central to developing and supporting good mental health [5]. Soon after he married in 1902, his new wife began visiting families of her husband's patients and her interest in the social environment profoundly influenced Meyer's work. Mental treatments, he argued, could not be considered apart from community structure. He argued that an ideal community should be rationally divided by districts so that complete households could be supported by access to political parties, access to police and health officers. Mental hospitals, within this plan, could be responsive to their districts with workers and clients taking an active part in community life. Meyer's work was somewhat of a progressive response to Social Darwinism but it replaced it with a static view of social organization. Society, for Meyer, was composed of households linked together through value consensus and a natural division of labor. Household units could be carved up into homogeneous districts to be watched over by humane authorities such as the police and the courts who, in turn, enforced the majority values in laws and regulations. Both the individual psyche and the social community, according to Meyer, thrived in this healthy condition of natural and harmonious relationships.

An alternative psychiatric theory of family and social relationships, one which lent itself to a dialectical model of structure and change, emerged in the first few decades of the century within the literature of the Freudian School of Psychiatry.

Within Freud's writing could be found a conservative instinct theory and an examination of universal categories of mind, as well as an exploration into the relationship between societal power relations and societal conflicts. Analysts throughout the 20th century recognized the contradictory themes in Freud, and sought to explain them. Brown, in his *Toward a Marxist Psychology* contended that psychoanalysis grew out of a response to a world threat of imperialism, workers' movements, familial changes (especially the conflict between Victorian bourgeoisie puritanism and Victorian proletarian sexual exploitation) as well as general changes in the capitalist view of human nature [6]. He suggested that Freud's static view of human nature aimed at increasing discipline among the work force [6, pp. 14-15]. In a similar vein, Reiff saw Freud legitimating the privatization of self, while redefining radicalism as an expression of neurosis [7]. Both of these authors stressed the conservative, reductionistic aspects of Freudianism.

The usefulness of Freudian psychology to the growth of monopoly capitalism was also explored by Berger who wrote that the idea of the unconscious, paralleled the splitting of the private from public life in the political economic structure [8]. Such a split served both the dominant mode of production and the profession of psychiatry. The identity crisis, according to Berger, resulting from this split, left the individual wondering which self was real and how to gain control over both private and public self. Berger ingeniously pointed out that the psychoanalyst could come to the aid of both selves since the analyst could, in one helping role, "assist the privatized suburbanite in the interior decorating of his(her) sophisticated psyche" and also "assist him(her) in dealing more effectively with the actual or potential trouble makers in the organization" [8]. Other 20th century thinkers explored the conflict implications of Freud's conceptualization of the dialectical relationships among personality elements — id, ego, and superego, as well as the relationship between social and personal organization. Freud's emphasis on sexual expression and his psychoanalysis were seen as direct challenges to the Victorian ethic.[1]

Followers of Freud also focused on bits and pieces of the master's work, developing their own psychologies and sociologies by elaborating on the basic Freudian framework. Reich for example, interpreted Freud's concept of repression as tacit agreement that human needs had to be curbed in the service of cultural and social development [9]. Reich's analysis of family structure as reflecting authoritarian State structure, and of repressed sexuality as serving capitalist production, exemplified the more radical interpretations of Freudian doctrine. The works of Norman O. Brown, Marcuse, and the Frankfurt School theorists further emphasized such conflict concepts within the Freudian School.

The social model of mental health and mental health illness which emerged from Freudianism was enhanced by attempts to synthesize Freudian psychology with sociological deviance theory. Early in the 20th century, U. S. social scientists eagerly joined the ranks of Freudians in developing the social side of the model. Anthropologists were especially enamored with the promise represented by Freud's special interest in cultural symbols. Pictures of Freud's study show it filled with exotic cultural artifacts from around the world, just one

[1] These themes can be found in the works of Norman O. Brown, R. L. Heilbroner, H. Marcuse, and W. Reich.

indication of his interest in what were considered primitive symbols of basic belief processes.

As Berger suggested, two propositions underscored this synthesis between the Freudian model of mind and of society, first the realization that a dialectical relationship existed between social structure and psychological reality, and second, that a dialectical relationship existed between psychological reality and prevailing psychological models [8]. The dialectic between society and the individual was spelled out by Freud in his sociological works on the relationship between individual repression and social order, for example, in *Civilization and Its Discontents* [10]. The message that civilization developed out of repression and out of neurosis rang all too true for persons who were experiencing the rapid removal of economic and political power from their own lives and away from their own communities during the rise of 20th century monopoly capitalism.

By the late 1920s and 1930s, the worldwide depression and its manifestation within the United States, especially the socialist labor movement, lent new urgency to theorizing on the social theory side of the mind-society synthesis. Some of the most influential societal elaborations came from ecological studies of deviance, pioneered by the University of Chicago which dominated sociological deviance studies. What had started during this period as studies of urban zones characterized by varying types and frequencies of deviance, during the following decades evolved into elaborate studies of the epidemiology of stress, class, and mobility. Such studies provided a common language linking medically training psychiatrists with academic social scientists. Social scientists such as Talcott Parsons (see Chapter 2) undertook psychoanalytic training and integrated this conservative Freudian perspective on mind into their unfolding analysis of social structure.

FROM FREUDING TO DRUGGING: 1940-1960

The Second World War provided a critical boost to the medicalization of deviance and to the profession of psychiatry. Large numbers of recruits from diverse ethnic and class backgrounds were suddenly defined as clients for psychiatric testing and treatment. Almost 2,000,000 were rejected from the military on the basis of psychiatric evaluations. Another 750,000 were discharged due to psychiatric problems [1, p. 57].

The importance of the War in building a coalition between nationally prominent psychiatrists, other mental health specialists and federal policymakers can hardly be overstated. Dr. Karl Menninger was appointed Chief of Army Psychiatry, Dr. Francis Braceland became Chief of Navy Psychiatry, and Dr. Robert Felix was Chief of the Public Health Service and the Coast Guard. These men were instrumental throughout the following decades in promoting the concept of community-based mental illness treatment based on what was known as public health psychiatry.

Medical schools began to institute abbreviated psychiatry training and to send new graduates out into the field for on-the-job experience. Within this wartime context, psychiatry could no longer depend for legitimation on the lengthy and costly treatment process of psychoanalysis. Mental health professional needed new theories and new treatments suitable to the military experience. Practitioners needed to return personnel to functional levels within short periods of time and at limited costs, a cost often borne by the federal government.

In the 1950s, psychiatry found a new core treatment in the development of drug therapy and the spread of so called brief treatments. The introduction of chlorpromazine (Thorazine) in the 1950s marked the start of a new efficient, medically dominated form of psychiatric/social control. Within eight months of its introduction by Smith, Kline and French, Thorazine had been given to an estimated 2,000,000 patients [11]. At the same time, state mental hospitals' in-patient populations were declining and the average length of stay were dramatically shortened.

By this period also, the medicalization of deviance had penetrated deeply into American culture, leading to what Miller and Reissman [12] called, "the psychiatric world view." According to these authors, by the late 1950s, psychiatry in the United States had successfully changed what formerly had been conceptualized as responsible choices and personal decisions into "unconsciously motivated acts." This conceptual innovation included the transformation of political and ideological views into the "authoritarian personality"; issues of crime and delinquency became problems of family instability or personality maladjustments; and political rebelliousness was defined away as a reflection of early parental relationships. Miller and Reissman wrote [12, p 204]:

> All kinds of problems—social, medical, educational, political—
> were interpreted through the new psychiatric world view. . . . This
> world view was costly in at least two ways: It deflected analysis and
> action away from non-psychodynamic (for example, social)

approaches and it often contaminated the original problem by introducing inappropriate modes of attack.

Obviously, despite drug treatment and short therapies, Freudianism continued to exert a significant influence on psychiatry, and it continued to reflect the works of both conservative consensual social scientists and conflict theorists. However, as medicalized models of mental illness continued to gain strength within the medical/ psychiatric arena, the dialectical content and critical tone inherent in the conflict language began to fall quickly from favor. The development of conflict social theory in the mental illness literature was dealt a near death blow during the era of McCarthyism and red-baiting when anything that could be termed communistic, including conflict sociology, became a dangerous topic for scholars worried about their jobs.

Another type of transformation in the development of social theory can be traced through the works of Frankfurt School authors who emigrated to the United States. Although conflict theoretical interpretations of Freud had been put forth rather vigorously in the pre-World War II, European works of the Frankfurt School authors such as Adorno, Horkheimer, and Marcuse, their later American works provided dramatic evidence of their acculturation to their new academic surroundings. The full impact of this change was explored by H. Stuart Hughes in his book, *The Sea Change: The Migration of Social Thought, 1930-1965* [13]. Hughes directed attention to the conservative influences which permeated the work produced by these authors in an intellectual community which was fascinated with models borrowed from the natural sciences and which were easily operationalized. Through these influences, the European conflict or prophetic tradition in social theory was being remodeled into priestly American consensualism. Along with this shift away from conflict theory, came a general diminishing of interest in the social side of psychiatry in the mainstream mental illness literature. Mental illness, increasingly became defined strictly in terms of biological, chemical or other such "hard science" approaches. Such approaches were not only more easily fundable as science but they also firmly legitimated psychiatry as a branch of medicine rather than a social science.

This shift was also mirrored in related fields such as psychology and social work. Psychological ego theorists elevated the rational component of mind, ego, as conceptualized by Freudians, to an independent status thereby implying the primacy of rationality in human motivation. Although psychologists were more likely to retain an interest in the social side of the mind-society synthesis, they also tended rather uncritically to adopt consensual approaches. In most of this literature, mental illness was conceptualized as individual maladjustments to the prevailing societal norms, values, and roles. For many ego psychologists, therapy was a tool for reintegrating non-conforming individuals into white, middle-class society.

One of the most interesting commentaries on this conservative bias within ego psychology was Russell Jacoby's *Social Amnesia: A Critique of Conformist Psychology from Adler to Laing* [14]. Jacoby focused his analysis on the forgetting of history in the service of conformist theory. He explored the radical interpretations of Freud, highlighting writings on unfulfilled human potential for liberation, the place of sexuality, pleasure, culture, and repression. Conservatism, he suggested, was built into neo-Freudianism, including the ego psychologies, by forgetting their earlier radical roots. It was conveniently forgotten that Freud stressed the possibility of liberating the self through dialectical struggle within the personality and within the society. Jacoby explained that [14, p. 33]:

> As Freud himself knew this was the cutting and revoluntionary edge of psychoanalysis: the refusal to accept social and individual values abstracted from the concrete struggle of men and women against themselves and nature. Here critical theory follows Freud: he is revolutionary in that his theory is critical and materialistic. Psychoanalysis pulls the shrouds off the ideology of values, norms and ethics which is the stuff of Adler and the post-Freudians. . . . The values that the neo- and post-Freudians esteem are pieces of history scrubbed clean of their carnal and visceral origins.

The sanitized values, norms, and ethics were also the stuff of mid-century social systems theorists. They, too, scrubbed norms, values, and ethics clean of history. Sociologists, for their part, also were only too glad to forget their conflict heritage and to build their static structural models of social systems on the foundations of white, middle-class norms and values.

In the sociological deviance literature, many approaches to non-normative behavior were being introduced including differential association theory in the later 1950s, theories of juvenile delinquency and studies in symbolic interactionism in the 1960s and 1970s. Paralleling these developments, research in the mental illness literature shifted from an emphasis on social class, urbanism and mental pathology to mental illness research dominated by structural-functional analysis.

Examples of this are the works of Faris and Dunham on urbanism and treated illness, and of Hollingshead and Redlich on class differences in treated mental illness [15].

Within these consensual deviance theories, nonconforming behavior was conceptualized in a variety of ways, for example, by Merton (See Chapter 2) as the misfit between cultural goals and social means to achieve those goals; by others as socialization to deviant subcultures; as undue social stress related to a host of variables such as class status, downward mobility, or urban living. Whatever the particular focus of the work, the background assumptions were quite similar—that society existed in its normal state as an integrated system held together by consensually agreed upon norms, values, and roles.

Stress and psychopathology reflected system dysfunctions and were to be minimized through correcting either the individuals' socialization or, at most, through redesigning some particular subsystem, such as a deviant subculture, within the total society. Stress and psychopathology were often traced to rapid social change, a condition which would be corrected with the reintegration of the various societal subsystems.

Symbolic interactional theorists and labelling theorists who came to the forefront of the literature in mid-decade emphasized the subjective perception of the world rather than material deprivation. As Gouldner wrote of one such theory, "Here men are not viewed as trying to do something but as trying to 'be' something" [16, p. 380]. Again by shifting their gaze away from the uncomfortable topics of class struggles, exploitation, and material deprivation, such social scientists were more easily able to undertake joint projects with their medical/psychiatric colleagues. The dialogue could be based on individual patients and their current symptomatology rather than on broader societal and historical processes.

CONFLICT AND CHANGE: THE LEGACY OF THE 1960s

By the 1960s, the medical model of mental illness with its implicit consensual social model, had many powerful supporters in the professions of psychiatry and psychology, and it was well integrated into mass culture. It also had considerable political support not only in voluntary associations such as the National Mental Health Association but also among politicians. The coalition among psychiatrists, federal policy-makers at the National Institute of Mental Health, and key Congressional figures, which had been forged during the Second World War, was stronger than ever. (See a fuller description in Chapter 4.)

In successive waves, the civil rights movement, anti-Vietnam War movement, and the women's movement flooded the American consciousness in the late 1950s gaining momentum through the 1960s. Worldwide, colonial rulers in Africa and Asia were being overthrown by nationalistic governments. Far reaching adjustments in the world system were manifested in anti-colonialist wars as well as through mass-based movements within the core capitalist nations. Student protesters in France and in the United States demanded control over their universities and their nation's policies. Issues of governmental social control versus individual autonomy dominated the news.

In the United States, the Vietnam wartime economy was fueling monopoly capitalism, and the accumulated economic surplus was being directed into social control efforts first targeted at the civil rights riots, then to larger areas of overt unrest.

Sociologists, meantime, both consensualists and conflict theorists, found new support in their attempt to elaborate the sociological side of the mind-society synthesis. Sociologists had been studying many facets of mental illness ranging from its definition to its treatment. The definition of mental illness had been expanding its boundaries so as to widen psychiatric territory almost without limit [17].

Community psychology had also made significant gains. Thanks largely to funding and direction from the federal government, training in psychology greatly expanded along with training in other mental health professions. According to Ozarin, in 1948 there were 1,500 psychologists working in mental hospitals [18]. By 1982, there were 27,000 psychologists with Ph.D.'s. This compares to 4,500 psychiatrists in 1948 and 30,000 by 1982.

The orientation of community psychology often reflected less of the individualistic medical model than did traditional medicalized psychiatry. Still, within its literature could be found a wide range of community approaches from the most conservative consensual to the more radical of the humanist psychologists. Thanks largely to the community orientation, ecological models became major conceptual tools for the mainstream of the discipline [19].

Radical social critics from medicine, psychology, sociology and other disciplines, emboldened by the activist atmosphere of the mid-to-late 1960s and the early 1970s, aimed their attacks at the very medical/psychiatric facilities which had invited them into their ranks a decade earlier. Ivan Illich explored the self-defeating implications of the medicalization of distress [20]. Vicente Navarro [21], Waitzkin and Waterman, Elliot Krause [23], and Alford [24] wrote on the relationships among infrastructural economic arrangements of the capitalist system in the United States and the role of medicine in social control. Analysts turned their attentions to which economic sectors reaped the most profits from existing medical/psychiatric arrangements, which sectors of other population were subjected to the heaviest social/psychiatric control and which aspects of mental illness treatment offered the most hope as emergent points of societal change.

On the international scene, psychiatry, which had formerly often been a welcome adjunct to the social control functions of colonial governments, was being attacked by angry critics. Franz Fanon, a young psychiatrist, radicalized during the Algerian War, roundly condemned psychiatric practice as a form of colonial domination [25]. In the United States, Grier and Cobbs insisted that much of what traditional psychiatry conceptualized as paranoid character traits among the black population, was the reflection of historically rooted rage at the contemporary black condition [26]. This critical attack organized itself into several major schools of thought including the anti-psychiatry movement, the feminist critique of psychiatry, and the community mental health literature.

ANTI-PSYCHIATRY

Anti-psychiatry was developed out of the writings and activity of a group of loosely connected critics whose common bond was chiefly their attack on the traditional medical model of mental illness and on traditional therapies. A typical example was *Realty Policy: The Experience of Insanity in America* by Brandt and published in 1975 [27]. Brandt's critiques of institutionalization focused on stigmatized public attitudes and abuses within institutions.

A prominent voice in this movement, E. Fuller Torrey, in his book, *The Death of Psychiatry* argued for the redefinition of traditional diagnostic categories from illness to "problems in living" [28]. To accompany this transformation, Torrey suggested a reconceptualization of what had been defined as therapy into what Torrey called educational courses in handling stress. In one form or another, the general message of most anti-psychiatry authors, was that the medical model of distress needed to be replaced with a new, but equally individualistic model.

Such thorough-going individualism was exemplified in the writing of another important anti-psychiatry author, equally heretical to traditional psychiatry but equally reductionistic in his approach, Thomas Szasz [29]. Szasz did not suggest a collectivistic approach to causation or cure. In place of the medical model, he espoused a rather nihilistic approach to distress, highlighting the social control functions of therapy.

In his landmark *Myth of Mental Illness* for example, Szasz decried the labelling of most mental illness as disease, but he failed to suggest a systematic alternative to the medical model [29]. Despite his scholarly analysis of the growth of psychiatry as a profession built upon the medical model and of psychiatry's social control role, the best Szasz could offer in place of traditional treatment was the suggestions that patients who felt the need for psychotherapy should be given the voluntary choice of treatment. The understanding by the patient of the therapist's social control function, in Szasz's view, was enough to legitimate the voluntary undertaking of treatment.

R. D. Laing, another major figure in the anti-psychiatry movement, sensitized his readers to an appreciation of altered states of consciousness. Laing argued in his works that individuals experienced such states for reasons understandable with the context of their own lives. In theory and in practice, Laing attempted to accept openly these experiences. Although he made an attempt to integrate this view within a larger political analysis of the role of mental illness and therapy in his master work, *The Politics of Experience* [30], at best his approach represented what sociologists were calling labelling or symbolic interactionism.

These anti-psychiatry authors vigorously criticized existing psychiatric practice but offered little consistent challenge to the political and economic role of psychiatry. Their reformist views on serving the economically disadvantaged sectors of society, or of treating individuals through more humane therapies underscored the romantic idealism which marked this literature. Such an approach was augmented by the outcries of politically active, often young radical authors. These writers attacked traditional practice from a thorough-going critique of its inherent sexism, elitism, and racism. (As will be shown in Chapter 5, many of these adopted a humanist marxist approach which developed within the CMHC literature.)

Radical Therapist, a journal published between 1970 and 1972, offered a forum for many of the more radical anti-psychiatry authors in this radical tradition. Although the journal was founded and initially guided by Michael Glen, a young psychiatrist serving in the Air Force in North Dakota during the Vietnam War, the journal eventually passed to control of a group called the Radical Therapy Collective formed in Boston. The Collective eventually changed the name of the journal to *Rough Times*, and then to *State and Mind*.

Many of the authors in this politicized wing of the anti-psychiatry movement had been inspired by, or had been active in a wide range of political causes in the late 1960s. Glen, for example, had been a psychiatric resident at the New York State Psychiatric Institute when he met Richard Kunnes, an activist resident at the same institute. Kunnes was active with the Black Panther Party and other radical movements of the times. His politics lent to his anti-psychiatry analysis a more well-developed political critique.

When Glen finished his psychiatric training at the institute and went into the Air Force, he, his wife, and another couple founded *Radical Therapist* as an attempt to express their own concerns about traditional psychiatry and to offer others an outlet for their concerns. After Glen finished his military service, he and most of the group moved to Cambridge, Massachusetts, and formed the nucleus of the Radical Therapy Collective. Only a year after its founding, the journal had a subscription list of over 20,000 names. Contributors to the journal, representing the diverse constituency of the anti-psychiatry movement, included California authors interested in human growth and potential, Lincoln Hospital activists from New York, who, like Kunnes, worked with the Black Panther Party, the Young Lords, an Hispanic group, other mass-based activist groups and leftist academics. The journal included articles on numerous liberation groups—gay rights, women's rights, mental patients' liberation, and anti-racism. It was the very existence of these groups that in a real way gave the anti-psychiatry movement its momentum, its audience, and its funding. In sum, it was the same political economic context which supported these groups and supported the anti-psychiatry movement, as will be shown in following chapters.

A review article by John Talbott, covering the original two year life span of *Radical Therapist*, summarized major topics in that journal and the radical anti-psychiatry movement in general [13]. According to Talbott, major topics in *Radical Therapist* were the political power of psychiatry, the importance of social and political action as therapy, community mental health as a rip-off, psychiatric oppression of minority groups and criticism of traditional individual therapies such as ECT and drugs. Talbott voiced standard criticism of the anti-psychiatry movement when he charged that although it espoused radical new directions, the theory and planning available from anti-psychiatry fell far short of a unified alternative. As summarized by

Talbott, the movement's chief theorists were closet traditionalists [31, p. 126].

> While Laing's view that craziness is creative may be radical, his psychoanalytic underpinnings, study of linguistics, and understanding of family dynamics are quite traditional. Similarly, Szasz may be in favor with the radicals for his opposition to the medical model, but his espousal of views applauded by reactionaries and his traditionally oriented one-to-one private psychoanalytic practice are hardly compatible with radical thought.

This lack of a unified alternative theory was acknowledged within the anti-psychiatry literature. As Talbott reported in 1977, one of the major contributors to the journal, Steiner developed a four-fold typology of therapies and their associated politics. In this typology, therapies were classified as either conventional/liberal or radical. Each of these two categories was paired with either conventional/liberal or radical politics. According to Steiner, only radical therapy and radical politics had no well-developed theory and therapy; radical political critiques had not produced parallel radical psychiatric theory. Even the conflict insights produced by Marcuse and others from the Frankfurt School tradition had given little sense of direction for a unified alternative to traditional approaches. Psychoanalysis did not seem an acceptable alternative, nor did the trendy techniques of Fritz Perls or Eric Berne, which were seen as disguised offshoots of traditional, liberal philosophies according to Steiner. Even the most non-traditional approaches such as those suggested by Timothy Leary and his psychedelic drug followers seemed to fail to move beyond romanticized calls for free love and personal liberation.

Perhaps mirroring the general disorganization of the anti-psychiatry movement, the Radical Therapy Collective which published the *Radical Therapist* itself fell victim to quarrels between members who supported one faction or another among the various social movements of the day. Factionalism within the membership ultimately led to the collective's demise in the mid-1970s. Indeed as will be discussed in the next chapter, the mid-1970s marked a turning point in the political economy of mental illness treatment, one characterized by a new brand of traditionalism.

Steiner himself was first author on an edited collection of writings from the West Coast counterpart of the Boston Radical Therapy Collective. The Berkeley, California collective was called the Radical Psychiatry Center, and their volume was entitled, *Readings in Radical*

Psychiatry, and was published in 1975. As the authors asserted [32, p. 159]:

> Liberation within an oppressive society is not possible. It is a mystification. People cannot be truly free if this society is not free because social oppression will necessarily impinge on their freedom.

The volume if filled with humanist talk of unequal power and oppression which characterized radical anti-psychiatry.

A practicing psychiatrist, Eileen Walkenstein, in 1976 published a poetry-filled attack on traditional psychiatric diagnosis and treatment. In *Don't Shrink To Fit! A Confrontation with Dehumanization in Psychiatry and Psychology*, Dr. Walkenstein shared her bitterness over traditional psychoanalytic approaches to what was termed mental illness, and her dissatisfaction with trendy alternative therapies such as bioenergetics, primal scream groups and offshoots of Frederick (Fritz) Perls' work [33]. In the tradition of anti-psychiatry the author wrote [33, p. 22]:

> A psychiatric diagnosis is like a jail sentence, a permanent mark on your record that follows you wherever you go. And even though psychiatrists know how little value there is in their diagnoses, they persist in playing Judge, handing down the sentences.

One of the most interesting insights offered in this particular work is the fact that clients of chic alternative therapies of the times became socialized to the language and behaviors associated with those therapies just as certainly as did believers in traditional treatments [33, p. 130]:

> Whereas in my previous psychiatric practice I could almost always tell, within a few minutes, which persons had subjected themselves to prior psychoanalytic treatment by automatic verbal analyzing and formulating, here in these 'Growth Center' groups I began to know which persons were the 'group' habitues. . . . The ready-made scream, the primal shout, the body heaving in pseudo-orgastic convulsions were as difficult a set of defenses against expressing the real human flow as the cerebral counterpart of those in the Freudian mold. These "groupies" had simply learned a new testament to replace the orthodoxy of the Freudian scripture.

Indeed subcultures built on such alternatives captured both popular and professional attention by the mid-1970s [34]. Anti-psychiatry created an unwelcomed sense of public skepticism directed toward the "priests" of mainstream mental illness treatment. In 1978, J. K. Wing, a student of prominent sociologist, David Mechanic, authored a work on social and political issues related to psychiatry [35]. Wing wrote of the anti-psychiatry movement [35, p. 231]:

> In recent years we have seen the development of an anti-psychiatry movement that carried considerable conviction, in spite of the lack of evidence for its more extreme assertions and strong body of evidence against them. That movement is now in disarray, perhaps because it tried both to destroy and to promise too much. The fantasies of revoluntionaries have tended, in our time, to be expressed in psychiatric (or anti-psychiatric) terms, just as, in the 17th century, they found expression in the form of religious (or anti-religious) experiences.

In fact, despite its lack of one unified political and ideological direction, anti-psychiatry did seem to be based more on various alternative sociopolitical and economic theories than on one alternative epistemology. In spite of their diverity, the messages voiced by its authors were alike in being thoroughly heretical to mainstream thinkers.

Inside even the most elite halls of psychiatry and inside medicine as a whole there was a new appreciation of the social control and political implications of therapy. No less a source than the *New England Journal of Medicine* published an article entitled, "Hidden Conceptual Models in Clinical Psychiatry" [36], in which the author, Lazare, traced the eclectic assortment of ideologies underlying psychiatric practice. A similar but more extensive review of models informing theories of mental illness was put forward by Siegler and Osmond in 1974 in their work, "Models of Madness, Models of Medicine" [37]. These authors identified eight models of psychiatric practice including medical models, moral models, psychoanalytic models, etc. Despite this seeming diversity, the individualistic and reductionistic underpinnings remained constant.

FEMINISM

Another main critique of traditional psychiatry during this mid-1960s emerged from the renewed vigor of the woman's movement. One of the major offshoots of the movement was a deep-seated concern with women's health care. As described by Sheryl Ruzek in her book, *The Women's Health Movement: Feminist Alternatives to Medical Control* [38, p. 60]:

Feminism exerted an influence on many social movements flourishing in the late 1960s, altering the directions of some movements and leading women to break away from the older, male-dominated movements. Women involved in the free clinic and radical health movements formed crucial initial constituencies of the women's health movement.

Feminists worked in the free clinic movement, the Medical Committee for Human Rights [39], the Health Policy Advisory Committee, and other activist groups of the 1960s. These women activists also formed an important constituency in the anti-psychiatry movement. The role of women in medical schools and in other prestigious mental health professions was criticized by feminists.

Elyse Zukerman complied an annotated bibliography of works on women and mental health [40]. In her *Changing Directions in the Treatment of Women: A Mental Health Bibliography*, Zukerman surveyed the extensive literature which had been developed out of women's mental health interest. Research covered issues from women as patients to women as practitioners. This literature, like that of anti-psychiatry, was strong on diversity and weak on unified alternatives to traditional psychiatric theory and therapies. Also lacking was a pragmatic political agenda through which to successfully challenge the traditional coalitions between politicians and members of the medical/psychiatry community.

COMMUNITY MENTAL HEALTH

Judged by the criterion of political viability, the most far-reaching movement within American psychiatry during these years was the community mental health centers (CMHC) movement. Community mental health found active support both among radical activists and mainstream traditionalists. Despite the fact that CMHC's were able to capture millions of dollars in federal funding through major acts of Congress, the movement was supported by some leaders of radical mass-based groups who usually opposed federal initiatives.

In addition to uniting extremely diverse political elements under its banner, the community mental health movement also reflected extremes of theory in its literature. Both conflict and consensus authors were represented in the CMHC literature. The uneasy synthesis between models of mind and models of society which had developed in the American psychiatric literature was newly synthesized in the CMHC movement. This movement not only brought academic theory into the realm of public policy, but it also united psychiatric and sociological professionals in joint theory building ventures, in policy, and in planning.

SUMMING UP

The history of the rise and fall of schools of thought in this uneasy synthesis between models of mind and models of society cannot be understood simply as paradigm shifts, schools growing or receding on the basis of the intellectual stimulation they offer to scholars. Rather, the assertion made here follows on the works of Gouldner and Friedrichs which suggest that each school carries with it specific background assumptions, often of an ideological nature. These assumptions mean that one theory will prosper while another will fail to attract attention based on its fit with the political economic needs of each historical period. This helps explain why conflict analyses of Freud could prosper in the European intellectual community of pre-World War II and virtually disappear in the post-War, American scholarly literature. The more individualistic and reductionistic the models of mind and of society, the more easily they translated into medical research.

As an introduction to later detailed analysis of the CMHC theory literature, it is useful to categorize some of the major schools addressed in this chapter. In Table 2, the sociological content of several major schools of social psychiatry theory is dichotomized into conflict and consensus theory. The psychiatric content is categorized by level and target of intervention. This creates a four cell figure.

Those schools of thought which most broadly support psychiatry as a medical specialty are located in cells 1 and 3. Cells 2 and 4 represent the conflict heritage of the American literature. Cell 4 contains schools of thought which have been described in this chapter as fragmentary conflict analysis, lacking a unified alternative to traditional theories and therapies.

Community mental health is not placed on this figure. It will be suggested in the following analysis that the CMHC literature cuts across levels of intervention and across sociological theories. This diversity makes the literature especially useful in analyzing the changing interest which theory serves.

Table 2. Fitting Schools of Social Psychiatry into
Types of Sociological Theory

| | | Sociological Content | |
		Consensus	Conflict
Level and Target of Intervention	Individual/ Medical	1 Social Darwinism Ego Psychology Conservative Freudianism	2 Radical Freudianism Frankfurt School
	Collective/ Social	3 Moral Treatment Adolf Meyer's Approach	4 Radical Anti-psychiatry Feminist Psychiatry

REFERENCES

1. P. Conrad and J. W. Schneider, *Deviance and Medicalization: From Badness to Sickness*, The C. V. Mosby Company, St. Louis, 1980.
2. R. Caplan, *Psychiatry and the Community in 19th Century America*, Basic Books, New York, 1969.
3. F. J. Braceland, *The Institute of Living*, The Institute of Living, Hartford, Connecticut, 1972.
4. B. Ehrenreich and D. English, *For Her Own Good: 150 Years of the Experts' Advise to Women*, Anchor Books, New York, 1979.
5. F. G. Alexander and S. T. Selesnick, *The History of Psychiatry: An Evaluation of Psychiatric Thought and Practice from Prehistoric Times to the Present*, Harper & Row, New York, pp. 262-265, 1966.
6. P. Brown, *Toward A Marxist Psychology*, Harper, New York, 1974.
7. P. Rieff, *Freud: The Mind of the Moralist*, University of Chicago Press, Chicago, 1959.
8. P. L. Berger, Toward a Sociological Understanding of Psychoanalysis, *Social Forces, 32*, 1965.
9. P. A. Robinson, *The Freudian Left*, Harper & Row, New York, pp. 11-73, 1969.
10. S. Freud, *Civilization and Its Discontents*, Anchor Books, New York, 1952.
11. T. P. Swazey, *Chlorpromazine in Psychiatry*, MIT Press, Cambridge, Massachusetts, 1974.
12. S. M. Miller and D. Riessman, *Social Class and Social Policy*, Basic Books, New York, 1968.

13. H. S. Hughes, *The Sea Change: The Migration of Social Thought, 1930-1965*, Harper & Row, New York, 1975.
14. R. Jacoby, *Social Amnesia: A Critique of Contemporary Psychology from Adler to Laing*, Beacon Press, Boston, 1975.
15. S. Cole, The Growth of Scientific Knowledge: Theories of Deviance as a Case Study, in *The Idea of Social Structure*, L. A. Coser (ed.), Harcourt Brace Jovanovich, Publishers, New York, 1975.
16. A. W. Gouldner, *The Coming Crisis of Western Sociology*, Basic Books, New York, 1970.
17. H. W. Dunham, Community Psychiatry: The Newest Therapeutic Bandwagon, *Archives of General Psychiatry*, pp. 303-313, 1965.
18. L. D. Ozarin, Community Mental Health: Does It Work?: Review of the Evaluation Literature, in *An Assessment of the Community Mental Health Movement*, W. Barten and C. Sanborn (eds.), Lexington Books, Lexington, Massachusetts, 1977.
19. J. G. Kelly, Ecological Constraints on Mental Health Services, *American Psychologist, 21*, pp. 535-539, 1966.
20. I. Illich, *Medical Nemesis: The Expropriation of Health*, Calder and Boyars, London, 1975.
21. V. Navarro, *Medicine under Capitalism*, Prodist, New York, 1976.
22. H. B. Waitzkin and B. Waterman, *The Exploitation of Illness in Capitalist Society*, Bobbs-Merrill, Indianapolis, 1974.
23. E. P. Krause, *Power and Illness: The Political Sociology of Health and Medical Care*, Elsevier, New York, 1977.
24. R. R. Alford, *Health Care Politics: Ideology and Interest Barriers to Reform*, University of Chicago Press, Chicago, 1975.
25. F. Fanon, *The Wretched of the Earth*, Grove Press, New York, 1968.
26. W. H. Grier and P. M. Cobbs, *Black Rage*, Bantam Books, New York, 1968.
27. A. Brandt, *Reality Police: The Experience of Insanity in America*, William Morrow and Company, Inc., New York, 1975.
28. E. F. Torrey, *The Death of Psychiatry*, Penguin Books, New York, 1974.
29. T. S. Szasz, *The Myth of Mental Illness*, Harper & Row, New York, 1961.
30. R. D. Laing, *The Politics of Experience*, Ballantine Books, New York, 1967.
31. J. A. Talbott, Radical Psychiatry: An Examination of the Issues, *American Journal of Psychiatry, 131*:2, pp. 121-128, 1974.
32. C. Steiner, H. Wyckoff, D. Goldstine, P. Lariviere, R. Schwebel, J. Marcus and members of the Radical Psychiatry Center (eds.) *Readings in Radical Psychiatry*, Grove Press, New York, 1975.
33. E. Walkerstein, *Don't Shrink to Fit: A Confrontation with Dehumanization in Psychiatry and Psychology*, Grove Press, New York, 1976.
34. P. Sedgwick, *Psycho Politics*, Harper & Row, New York, 1982.
35. J. K. Wing, *Reasoning about Madness*, Oxford University Press, New York, 1978.

36. A. Lazare, Hidden Conceptual Models in Clinical Psychiatry, *New England Journal of Medicine, 288*, pp. 345-351, 1973.
37. M. Siegler and H. Osmond, *Models of Madness, Models of Mind*, Harper & Row, New York, 1974.
38. S. B. Ruzek, *The Woman's Health Movement: Feminist Alternatives to Medical Control*, Praeger Press, New York, 1978.
39. L. S. Linn, Physician Characteristics and Attitudes toward Legitimate Use of Psychotherapeutic Drugs, *Journal of Health and Social Behavior, 12*, pp. 132-141, 1971.
40. E. Zukerman, *Changing Directions in the Treatment Women: A Mental Health Bibliography,*, NIMH, Rockville, Maryland, 1979.

CHAPTER 4

The Political Economy and the Community Mental Health Movement

What were the forces in the larger political economic context which limited and guided the development of social psychiatric theory? In the preceding chapter, social psychiatry was shown to have developed as a combination of models of mind and of society. This uneasy combination reflected events internal to specific disciplines and events in the wider society.

In the current chapter, that wider society will be explored in terms of the State and the economy.[1] The economy includes the capitalist marketplace. The chapter begins with an overview of the movement, moves to the specific model of the political economy adopted for this analysis, and continues with a discussion of the movement in its three distinct political economic phases.

AN OVERVIEW OF THE MOVEMENT: REVOLUTION OF EVOLUTION?

Authors writing in the early phase of the CMHC movement vividly expressed the enthusiasm which many felt regarding this promised

---

[1] State with a capital "S" refers to the overall governmental form, while "state" with a small "s" refers to an individual state as the state of New York.

"bold new approach" to mental health care. Bellak one of the leaders of community psychiatry, wrote in his oft-cited article, "Community Psychiatry: The Third Psychiatric Revolution," that the community psychiatry component of the CMHC movement represented a third revolution for the profession, the first two being moral treatment and Freudianism [1]. By 1974, however, this same author had muted his assessment to that of evolution rather than revolution. To paraphrase Bloom, a noted social psychologist, the CMHC movement was part of a larger revolution of social responsibility that included the civil rights movement, education and voting rights; part of a geo-political revolution that had resulted in the establishment of the local community as a unit important enough to receive the direct attention of the federal government; part of a planning revolution; part of a citizens' participation revolution; and part of a revolution in the prevention of poverty, physical disability, malnutrition, and under education [2]. No small claim for one legislative program.

Opposing these lofty sentiments were those who berated the movement as little more than the expansion of professional turf. Rieff wrote that, far from revolution, community mental health was really an [3, p. 60]: . . . extension of current professional ideology with modified goals, tactics and technologies over that part of society from which it has been hitherto alienated; (that it is a consolidated system of care which) legitimates a two-class system of mental health treatment in this country—self-actualization for the rich, rehabilitation for the poor. The 1974 Nader Report on the movement, by Chu and Trotter [4] summed up its review of the movement by entitling one of its final chapters, "Innovation Without Change."

The explanation for this cooling of initial enthusiasm can be found in the roots of the movement itself. The movement began not as a mass-based social movement, but as a movement on many levels. In one sense, it began with a relatively small coalition of public health psychiatrists and federal administrators. Once underway, it underwent important changes which reflected various State functions which it served, and various market conditions to which it reacted. This is not to argue that such were the intentions of the major figures in the movement. Many, if not most, were undoubtedly well-meaning professionals in their various fields who sought to make good mental health care more readily available to the many who needed help. Nonetheless, when looked at from a higher level of abstraction, a sociological level, the movement as a whole can be seen as serving State and market functions.

The policy to shift persons out of state hospitals and into "community" facilities caught the scholarly attention of social scientists throughout the 1960s and 1970s, as will be shown in this and the following chapters. Two penetrating analyses which focused attention on the underlying political economic implications of this move were authored by Scull [5] and Brown [6].

The first was a landmark work entitled, *Decarceration*, authored in 1977 by Andrew Scull. In this work, Scull documented how persons labeled deviant were moved out of state funded long-term care facilities into welfare hotels or were simply dumped on the streets in the mental health reform. Scull wrote [5, p. 152]:

> Placing the decarceration movement in historical context, I have argued that this shift in social control styles and practices must be viewed as dependent upon and a reflection of more extensive and deep-seated changes in the social organization of advanced Capitalist societies. In particular, it reflects the structural pressures to curtail sharply the costly system of segregative control once welfare payments, providing a subsistence existence for elements of the surplus population, make available a viable alternative to management in an institution. Such structural pressures are greatly intensified by the fiscal crisis encountered in varying degrees at different levels of the state apparatus; a crisis engendered by advanced capitalism's need to socialize more and more of the costs of production—the welfare system itself being one aspect of this process of socialization of costs.

Indeed, the tremendous increase in welfare payments and the structural changes in the mental illness treatment market did have the impact of transferring costs from states to the State. This was further articulated by Brown.

Brown focused attention on how and why the cost of mental illness care was transferred to the federal government. He located the causes of this transfer in three major structural forces—1) political economic factors, 2) professionalist forces, and 3) institutional factors at the level of the psychiatric system and individual facilities. For the first, emphasis was placed on the profit motive driving care, State financing such as Medicare and Medicaid, the role of health care in reinforcing and replicating existing class, gender and race stratification, and the fragmented nature of the care [6, pp. 10-11]. Professional forces created the expansion of the psychiatric domain within everyday life. Regarding the third element, institutional factors, Brown looked at the creation of national policy which resulted from the strong lobbying efforts on behalf of mental institutions, as well as the problems dealt with by individual mental institutions including charges of custodialism and the reactions to it such as those from the anti-psychiatry forces. Brown's analysis focused needed attention on the "new alliances" of public and private sectors, private mental hospitals and general hospital psychiatric units. He also added innovative material on the patient's rights movement and homelessness among ex-mental patients.

The fiscal pressures explicated by Scull and Brown must be considered along with such elements as employment trends [7, 8] the treatment trends discussed in Chapter 7, as well as the momentum generated by the theory addressed in the latter part of this book.

The next section will expand on the economic and political underpinnings by detailing distinct phases in the CMHC movement. The parallel between these political economic eras and the application of the concept of community during each will provide the threads from which the remainder of the book is woven.

ELEMENTS OF THE POLITICAL ECONOMY

The CMHC movement was very much a product of the federal government, but it must be understood within the context of the State in general. It served and responded to not only federal needs, but also to local and state governments. One of the functions it served was that of social control for the State, in this way ideological control was balanced off against the raw force of police and military might which was also at the State's disposal. Certainly resocialization of "deviants" through mental illness treatment and social investment in political trouble spots were less controversial means of social control than were police and military intervention.

In order to better understand how such control served the State, it is necessary to understand what the concept of State functions includes. Mandel presented a model of State functions which bridged earlier gaps in State theory [9]. Rather than conceptualize the State as purely an instrument of one dominant class (instrumental theory), or as purely the outcome of structural processes of the State (structuralist theory), Mandel portrayed the State as incorporating a variety of functions which at times responded to the dominant class, and at times served the processes of class struggle. Mandel saw the State as fulfilling at least the following functions [9, p. 475]:

i) Provision of those general conditions of production which cannot be assured by the private activities of the dominant class.

ii) Repression of any threat to the prevailing mode of production from the dominated classes or particular sections of the dominated classes, by means of army, police, judiciary and prison system.

iii) Integration of the dominated classes, to ensure that the ruling ideology of society remains that of the ruling class, and that consequently the exploited classes accept their own exploitation with the immediate exercise of the repression against them (because they believe it to be inevitable, or the "lesser evil," or "superior might"or fail even to perceive it as exploitation).

In these ways, the State acted both to secure continued accumulation for the dominant political economic interests, and to legitimate dominant ideological control. The CMHC movement fit these functions, in part, by 1) extending the material infrastructure of the mental illness treatment marketplace, 2) providing effective State social control beyond that accomplished by the threat of police and military force, and 3) supporting the existing cultural dominance.

Mandel's State model fills in the "political" side of the political economic equation for the current analysis. The economic side is addressed nicely in O'Connor's *Fiscal Crisis of the State* [10, 11]. O'Connor divided the market into three interlocking sectors—State, monopoly, and competitive. O'Connor agreed with Mandel that the State mediated among classes in order to sustain accumulation and to legitimate the capitalist system as a whole.

O'Connor went beyond Mandel in exploring how the market functioned to support these State functions. According to O'Connor, each of the three sectors of the market was characterized by such features as the ratio between capital intensity and labor intensity (i.e., the investment in machinery versus investment in human labor power), the size of the production market, and the insulation of the sector from fluctuation in labor demand. The monopoly sector was capital intensive, produced for large markets, and had stable labor demand. The competitive sector was labor intensive, produced for small markets, and had variable labor demand. The State sector varied, depending on its role in controlling the overall market.

Although contradictions among and within sectors exerted significant influence on the overall State-market relationship, in the long run, major groups in the monopoly sector used publicly financed infrastructural arrangements to support their own privatized monopoly sector profits.

The State also provided public support for a variety of social programs in order to control the workforce and to assure continuation of the market. Factions within the State acted to preserve high rates of profit for the monopoly sector—profits which were produced from the publicly supported infrastructure such as roads, communication, and publicly financed buildings. As competition and expansion within the market increased, so too, socialized costs increased in order to sustain the infrastructure for these high levels of privatized, monopoly profits. The process was inherently inflationary and ultimately produced what O'Connor called the fiscal crisis of the State [10].

Psychiatrists, as other M. D.s, were not structurally part of the monopoly sector in the same way as were the drug and hospital corporate entities. Nonetheless, they did share the same market interests to a considerable extent. Psychiatrists acted to enlarge their market and to sustain significant control over what historically had been defined as their professional domain. The State underwrote the costs of much of their market expansion through the CMHC movement. This is not to imply that a conspiracy existed between medical/psychiatric interests and political ones. Rather, the mental illness treatment needs of the nation were defined by public health psychiatrists and their colleagues in a way that led public officials to feel that they were responding to objective needs. Whether they were or were not is a question beyond the scope of the present analysis. The major point here is simply that professionals who controlled the market and who chiefly benefited from its expansion, were able to convince public officials to underwrite large portions of the market expansion through the outlay of public funds. The emphasis here is placed on psychiatry rather than on other mental health disciplines because most of the political and economic impetus for the CMHC movement revolved around that discipline. Public health and community psychologists did play a notable role in concert with psychiatrists, and their theory will be included in the following chapters.

Table 3 summarizes market trends, State functions, and legislation in each of the three CMHC movement phases to be discussed.

PHASE I. INFRASTRUCTURE EXPANSION AND TARGETED CONTROL

As early as the 1930s, the basis was being laid for the community mental health model of service delivery. The theory was called public health psychiatry (as mentioned in the previous chapter)

Table 3. Summary of State, Market, and Legislation during the Three Major Phases
of the Community Mental Health Movement

Period	Market	State Functions	Legislation and Regulations
Period I: late 1950s to mid-1960s	Market infrastructure expanded through federal monies. Monopoly sector in control.	Accumulated surplus expended. Force targeted at urban areas. Mental health and social services seen as ideological control.	Initial CMHC legislation and regulations passed. Five services are mandated.
Period II: mid-1960s to early 1970s	Infrastructure expansion continues with federal monies. Division of labor articulated. Competitive sector drawn into market.	Force widened to more diverse groups. Factions form around traditionalists and "radicals."	CMHC legislation renewed with expanded funding. Children and addicts added as target populations.
Period III: early 1970s to 1980	Market stabilizes. Funding emphasis switched to states and private sector.	Political support weakens. Special interest groups consolidate lobbying.	New planning schemes define consumers and providers. Evaluation emphasized. Carter administration produces President's Commission Report and Mental Health Systems Act.
Aftermath 1980 to 1990	Market fragments into public and private, good and poor payment sources.	Impetus returned to state governments and private sector.	Reagan block grants replace CMHC funding. Most federal money withdrawn.

59

and it was tied to a service delivery model based on local clinics in each community.

The public health view encompassed elements of individual vulnerability to illness, environmental characteristics which promoted or undercut the spread of illness, and agents of illness [12]. Although this view incorporated a societal model, it wedded it to the medicalized view of distress. The legacy of the asylum movement, and the spreading freudian influence, dominated the small but growing domain of psychiatry and psychology. Various other movements such as the child guidance movement of the 1920s, and the neighborhood health clinic movement helped mobilize public support for the enlargement of the role of public health experts in issues of mental well-being.

One of the fathers of the movement was Erick Lindemann, later known chiefly for his pioneering work on grief reactions, and crisis intervention. Lindemann, working with the Wellesley Human Relations Service Project in Wellesley, Massachusetts, with the Harvard Department of Social Relations, and as Chief of Psychiatry at the Massachusetts General Hospital, was instrumental in socializing a generation of influential mental health workers in the theory of early prevention and early intervention. He also established one of the first community mental health centers a decade before the federal legislation was passed. This center included not only the principles of good public health psychiatry, but the idea of consultation to front line mental health workers such as the clergy, nurses, and even bartenders.

Others working within the public health tradition included Robert Felix (later to found and expand the National Institute of Mental Health), who grew up in Kansas with two other key figures—William and Karl Menning [13].

Karl Menninger, one of the outstanding spokespersons for public health psychiatry, founded the American Orthopsychiatry Association [14, p. 57] and devoted his professional services to popularizing public health psychiatry. Using the language of public health, the legitimate domain of psychiatry was expanded, for example to schools, the legal system, and to religion.

In 1930, the first International Congress on Mental Hygiene helped form a Division of Mental Hygiene in the U.S. Public Health Service. Only eight years later, Laurence Kalb, a leader in public health psychiatry, took over the Division and built a stronghold for psychiatry in the National Institutes of Health.

Also in 1930, the Rockefeller Foundation financed a national mental hospital inspection program and began to lobby intensively for federal funding to improve conditions and staffing in these facilities. The Rockefeller Foundation was often active in the more general Western capitalist medical marketplace, working to expand it both nationally and internationally [15]. The Foundation, as part of this program, sponsored travelling fellowships for U.S. medical students interested in European medical study. (One of the recipients of this fellowship was Francis Braceland, later to become one of the founders of the CMHC movement.) The Rockefeller activities tended to catalyze liberal reformist crusades against custodial state hospital care, but they never challenged the fundamental medicalized/psychiatric theory behind such care.

The creation of the National Institute of Mental Health, in 1946, within the Public Health Service marked a formal shift in federal mental health policy away from narrowly defined service markets, such as the military, and toward increased federal intervention into the general service market. The newly created NIMH was mandated only to support research on issues of mental illness, to provide limited training, and small demonstration projects. Initially, it was only given one avenue of direct service in the form of aid and personnel from the Public Health Service for individual state government assistance.

Dr. Robert Felix, director of NIMH from its creation until 1964, was an especially strong advocate of the public health approach to psychiatry. He felt that the profession should include prevention, out-patient services, geographically responsible care, community involvement, and rational planning [16]. These principles, later to become extremely important in the CMHC literature, were first applied under federal direction through NIMH supported community mental health clinics in the 1940s and early 1950s. Tax supported clinics represented the first major entry by the federal government into direct services. As Connery et al. reported, of the 1234 tax supported clinics operating by 1954, almost 66 percent had been opened on or after the founding of NIMH [17]. Federally supported clinics increased the already close connection between advocates for psychiatry in voluntary special interest organizations and officials of the federal government. As the federal advocates gained strength within the bureaucracy, these interests also organized. By 1950, the National Committee merged with the National Mental Health Foundation and the Psychiatry Foundation, all public sector interest groups, to form the powerful National Association for Mental Health [18].

In the mid 1950s, federal mental health policy was being written by a small group of federal administrators, and being supported by social science research which explored the relationship between social factors and mental illness. The rise of consensual deviance theory provided a boost, rather than a challenge to the spread of medicalized services.

Although mental illness was recognized as a serious national issue after the shell shock cases of World War I, the need for services seemed to fade from the national consciousness after the War. As noted in the last chapter, World War II provided a new impetus to the expansion of the mental illness marketplace. The War mandated psychiatric evaluations for recruits, many of whom were rejected on the basis of the results. Somewhat to the surprise of those who planned the testing, such weeding out did not eliminate widespread mental health problems related to battle. In addition, many physicians were sensitized to the need for psychiatric skills in dealing with their patient population during and after the War. As a result, the Menningers turned a large hospital in Kansas into a Veterans Hospital which took on one hundred psychiatric residents rather than the usual two or three found in most hospitals.

The founders of NIMH were public health officers who "had matured in the atmosphere of World War II psychiatric success," who had classic psychiatric training, and who worked with a small number of interested officials in Congress, the National Committee Against Mental Illness, a few state mental health directors and a few professional social scientists and psychiatrists [19, p. 6]. Although, at first, in the early 1950s, NIMH's political battles were relatively small and localized inside the agency, by 1954, with more and more lay people and social scientists involved, NIMH had expanded into the realm of big business. Next to the Department of Defense, NIMH had become the largest supporter of behavioral scientists in the country [19, p. 9].

The War catalyzed much of this growth. The federal psychiatric leaders already inside the bureaucracy were able to increase their numbers. Dr. Robert Felix, Chief Psychiatrist in the Public Health Service, was also head of psychiatry for the Coast Guard. Chief of Navy Psychiatry was Dr. Francis Braceland, an advocate, along with Drs. Felix and Menninger, of federal support for increased availability of high quality psychiatry services in the community. These men met and worked closely during the war, forming coalitions which were to last well into the next decade.

During the same period, psychoanalytic institutes in several metropolitan areas such as Boston, Philadelphia, New York, and Washington were providing training grounds and meeting places for academic psychiatrists and a few social science colleagues. For example, the Boston Institute's first fellowship to a social scientist went to Louisa Howe in 1941, a sociologist who worked with the Menningers, Lindemann, and later Bertram Brown. Talcott Parsons was the Institute's second fellowship winner. The social science psychiatry connection was strengthened through the networks formed in these working relationship. Academic personnel working at Harvard and Brown, for example, were to take active roles in uniting federal initiatives with university interests during the CMHC movement.

The 1950s were crucial years for the expansion of public mental health policy. Foley and Sharfstein referred to the years 1946-1960 as those when mental health professionals were learning the political arts [20]. Indeed, it was in the early 1950s that the census of state hospitals began their long decline, which continues to the present day; 1955 was the year in which Congress passed legislation mandating NIMH to provide demonstration grants to state hospitals and it was the year of Public Law 84-182—the Mental Health Study Act [2, pp. 23-25]. The first two events paved the way for extended federal ventures into direct service provision; the third provided the vehicle for consolidation of public and private sector support for these ventures.

FEDERAL RESEARCH AS THE BASIS FOR FEDERAL ACTION

One of the most detailed historical accounts of the federal role in the creation of the CMHC legislation and its aftermath is found in Foley and Sharfstein [20]. This fascinating look begins with a listing of "key institutional players" including eleven departments of the federal government and eighteen special interest groups [20, p. xvii]. Its chronology of events begins with the 1854 veto by President Franklin Pierce of a bill which would have built public asylums at federal expense and ends with the 1981 Omnibus Budget Reconciliation Act which repealed most of the current mental health legislation in favor of block grants to states.

With regard to recent history, most authors agree that a key to the final passage of the CMHC legislation was the initiation of the Mental Health Study Act. In 1955, Congress mandated this Act, a five-year study funded by roughly $1,000,000 in federal support, plus about $140,000 in private support donated through twenty-one professional and business organizations. These latter represented a host of corporate and psychiatric interests. The list of participants and sponsors included the American Medical Association, the American Psychiatric

Association, the National Association for Mental Health, the Rocke-feller Brothers Fund, and the Smith, Kline and French Foundation. This can be interpreted as the time when the monopoly sector was organizing and forming coalitions between professionals and corporate interest, as well as between key personnel in the public and private sectors.

Prominent among individual participants in the study were Dr. Braceland, who was by then president of the American Psychiatric Association; Mike Gorman, long time prominent figure in the National Committee Against Mental Illness; Dr. Nicholas Hobbs from the American Psychological Association; and Dr. Jack Ewalt, Professor of Psychiatry at Harvard. These and other authors of the study repre-sented the links between academe, private interest groups, and cor-porate interests. Dr. Braceland and the study director, Dr. W. Appel, represented traditionally trained psychiatrists who were perceived as respected advocates for upgrading mental illness treatment services and for extending treatment sites to the community. Gorman and Hobbs represented public health psychiatrists who also were suppor-tive of treatment reform and the establishment of local clinics. Dr. Ewalt added an academic dimension, along with the prestigious Harvard connection. Dr. Ewalt was commissioner of the Mas-sachusetts Department of Mental Health, and was named director of the study staff of 60. In addition to work by full-time staff, ap-proximately 100 consultants were called upon during the course of the study. The product prepared by this Joint Commission on Men-tal Health was a report, *Action for Mental Health*, published in 1961, along with seven accompanying volumes dealing with a variety of issues from psychiatric facilities to training needs. The report, likened in impact to the Flexner Report which catalyzed reform of medical training earlier in the century, focused Congressional, as well as national, attention on reform of state hospitals [17, p. 37]. It suggested that community based clinics be linked to hospitals in order to decentralize and to improve care. Along with this plan came extensive reporting on the need to expand the labor pool for delivering mental illness treatment.

The authors of the report were writing in a time, the 1950s, when the mental illness treatment market provided about 1.7 million care episodes a year, with most treatment occurring in state hospitals, country hospitals, or general hospitals [21, p. 78]. In the 1950s, the direct costs of mental illness were estimated to be about $685,000,000 paid for by individual states; $322,000,000 paid for by the federal government, including $35,000,000 in support for NIMH; and another $179,000,000 covered by foundations, voluntary hospitals and private psychiatry [22, p. 46]. The states were increasingly anxious to shift costs to alternative sources of support. Psychiatry's interests were in market expansion, and federal officials held out hope that the post-War economy offered the economic potential for increased federal expenditures.

With these interests in mind, the authors of the Congressional study decried the low national priority assigned to mental health both in the public consciousness and in the federal budget. They included reference to the relatively small amounts for mental health raised by the public sector groups such as the National Association for Mental Health. Clearly such groups were as supportive of service expansion as were the professionals and the corporate interests. The study authors repeatedly stressed what they felt to be the tremendous national problem of mental illness, a problem vividly bought to the nation's attention during the War.

Study recommendations included increased research support and hospitals linked to community programs which would train caring persons to work in mental illness treatment. General hospital psychiatric units, units in small state hospitals, acute care centers and aftercare and rehabilitation units were all mentioned in the report. The Study Commission recommended that state, federal, and local expenditures for mental illness treatment be doubled in five years. In addition, it was suggested that Congress and NIMH should develop a federal subsidy program to encourage state and local governments to emulate VA hospitals in their psychiatric care, care which emphasized outpatient treatment and aftercare. These were elements of the mental illness treatment market which held a central place in the model of public health psychiatry.

At the same time that the Joint Commission was drawing up its report under a mandate from congress, the Surgeon General appointed his own committee to study needs and to assist states with developing comprehensive state mental health plans. According to Musto [16, p. 62]:

> The Committee's report stressed the need for many of the services that the Commission had mentioned, and favored even more stringent limits on the size of state mental hospitals. The federal legislation contemplated by the Committee also featured (as did the Commission's plan) federal funding through states, presumably for construction rather than staffing. Increased aid to the mentally ill

themselves was to come through public assistance provisions for the State Social Security Act. The Committee recognized the shortage of mental health professionals but pointed to the rapid growth in their numbers and claimed that good facilities in the rural areas proved themselves helpful in attracting competent medical personnel.

NIMH saw some key authors of the reports as bureaucrats, the same bureaucrats who had earlier authored the Hill Burton legislation which had used federal funds for the building of community hospitals throughout the country, but who were unprepared for innovative care. Many of the non-elite non-psychiatric authors were pictured as overly concerned with issues of administration and as lacking appropriate regard for psychiatric experts and their role. Some members of Congress and the Surgeon General were seen as supporting an NIMH model in which professionals controlled the research, and bureaucrats controlled the administrative dealings with the states on issues of service delivery [16, p. 63]. This fight between bureaucratic control and professional autonomy over mental illness care was to surface again in the late 1960s.

The immediate outcome was that NIMH developed its own report which, rather than focusing on a revised state hospital system, stressed the need for a community model including a series of 2,000 community mental health centers under psychiatric control. The authors of the NIMH report also suggested that rather than federal money going solely for construction of such centers, that federal support also should be allocated for staffing since too few trained personnel were currently available in the service market.

The psychiatric interests found a sympathetic supporter in President Kennedy, a man whose own family had experienced problems of mental illness and mental retardation. In 1963, President Kennedy appointed his own interagency committee to study each report and to suggest legislative action. The debates between state hospital reform and community mental health centers, between construction alone and construction plus staffing, between community and non-community models of care were largely resolved in NIMH's favor. Dr. Felix had won an important political victory.

In 1963, President Kennedy sent a message on mental health and mental retardation to Congress. This message included support of community mental health centers with both construction and staffing funds to cover 75 percent of total costs, stepped down over four years. In addition, state hospitals were to receive $10,000,000 to improve facilities and care—a concession to the powerful interests who backed state facilities.

KENNEDY'S MESSAGE

Kennedy began his message with a description of care in the country. He reported that 800,000 patients resided in the nation's psychiatric institutions, 600,000 of whom were mental patients; the rest being retarded. Each year, 1,500,000 cases received treatment in these institutions. The average amount spent on care per day was only $4.00; in some states it was as low as $2.00. Kennedy charged that most of these institutions were overcrowded, antiquated, and custodial in nature. Despite this, the cost to the taxpayers was more than 2.4 billion dollars a year, and indirect costs were much higher.

He noted that the federal government had traditionally left the issue of mental health care to the states and that the states had depended on custodial care and care in homes which were overcrowded and unpleasant. In one of the most frequently quoted passages from his message, Kennedy announced, "The time has come for a bold new approach" [23, p. 2]. This approach was to be based on new medical, scientific, and social treatment methods.

Kennedy's plan was to join federal, state and local governments in a three-pronged attack. First was prevention through seeking the causes and [23, p. 3]:

> The general strengthening of our fundamental community, social welfare, and educational programs which can do much to eliminate or correct the harsh environmental conditions which are associated with mental retardation and mental illness.

This compelling vision translated into expansion of medicalized psychiatric care into local clinic settings, school, social agencies, and the courts. Second was strengthening knowledge about training and manpower needs including professional and subprofessional personnel, and also including national service corps and youth employment training. Third was strengthening and improving programs and facilities which emphasized diagnosis, treatment, training, and rehabilitation. Federal money was to be used to stimulate state, local, and private action on all points.

Kennedy repeatedly called forth images of "the community." "When carried out, reliance on the cold mercy of custodial isolation will be supplanted by the open warmth of community concerns and capability"

[23, p. 3]. Thanks to treatment by drugs and to community care in general hospitals, day-care centers, and out-patient clinics, the state hospitals would fade away. "These Centers will focus community resources and provide better community facilities for all aspects of mental health care," [23, p. 5]. Being located in the patient's own environment, own community, the center would make possible a better understanding of needs, a more cordial atmosphere for recovery, and a continuum of treatment.

The use of the terms professionals and subprofessionals was a telling choice of words, reflecting as it did the continuing dominance of psychiatric and medical interests in this early plan for services. Nonetheless, many psychiatrists feared these services would dilute their control. Kennedy called for a new type of facility, ". . . one which returns mental health care to the mainstream of American medicine, and at the same time upgrades mental health services" [23, p. 5]. Here again the message to psychiatrists was not to worry about outside meddling in their professional domain. In addition, he called for private physicians, including general practitioners and psychiatrists to participate directly in the centers. Centers would provide auxiliary staff which private practitioners would use to treat their own patients [23, p. 4]. Clearly the support of the medical establishment in the passage of the legislation was to be crucial.

THE LEGISLATION

Success in meeting these goals and their translation into legislation depended largely on NIMH and its director, Dr. Felix, working in concert with key politicians in Congress. Three key political figures included Senator Lister Hill (D. Alabama), a longtime supporter of mental health legislation, Rep. John Fogarty (D., Rhode Island), and Rep. Oren Harris (D., Arkansas). A long parade of supporters passed before the Senate panel during their CMHC hearings on March 5, 6, and 7, 1963. On the first day of Congressional testimony, Dr. Felix, Dr. Ewalt, and Mike Gorman spoke in favor of the plan. First in line the second day came Dr. Braceland, representing the American Psychiatric Association; Dr. Hudson, from the American Medical Association; Dr. Hobbs, from the American Psychological Association, among others. The hearings were carefully orchestrated to shower praise on the program from elite representatives of medicine, psychiatry, associated groups in psychology, voluntary associations and others supporting the mental illness treatment market.

Major negotiations among public interest groups, private sector physicians, and state hospital interests had been carried out long before these Congressional hearings. In fact, the only issues which managed to surface in the hearings were: 1) the role of the state hospitals in the new scheme, and 2) the advisability of staffing grants. The role of state hospitals was addressed in testimony vividly recounting the inadequacies of care. Again and again the Congressmen heard the call to minimize the state hospital role in care. The issue of staffing grants was hotly contested. Some traditional medical interests called federal staffing grants "unnecessary" and an ill-advised intrusion of government into professional practice. The American Medical Association lobbied most extensively against the grants. Their fear was that if NIMH could pay the salaries of the CMHC staff, then the federal government could control professional medical/psychiatric practice. Eventually the Public Health and Safety Committee of the Senate cut funding for the proposal from 657 million to 284 million dollars. The House Committee on Interstate and Foreign Commerce eliminated the staffing grants completely, a victory for the American Medical Association.

The CMHC Act, which was passed in 1963, contained no provision for staffing grants, and contained less money than had been requested for construction. Nonetheless, it did establish the basis for a federally sponsored system of care in community based health centers. The legislation mandated coordinated, geographically focused treatment centers which were to be regionally planned and oriented toward prevention. The centers were to be composed of a set of comprehensive services which would initially be largely funded by the federal government.

Despite this legislation, the implementation and interpretation of the scheme had far to go. In fact, even while legislative and psychiatric leaders were congratulating themselves on their victory, problems were emerging with the legislation's implementation. One of the earlier problems to surface, and ultimately one of the most devastating quarrels, concerned the role of the states in the process of community care. For example, the Congress had appropriated 4.2 million in fiscal 1963 for states to draw up plans for mental health services. The funds were to be spent over the next two years in assisting states to develop their plans. Less than four months later, the CMHC legislation was enacted, authorizing funding before states could draw up plans. Many centers had to move quickly to negotiate places in partially prepared state plans. The virtual exclusion of state governments from the Act, and the direct funding of centers by the federal government was to prove a key factor in the CMHC movement. As will be shown later, the CMHC Act could be seen as just one of a number of federal initiatives into local communities which bypassed state governments during the Kennedy era.

The assassination of President Kennedy brought into office a new President, and renewed Congressional resolve to carry through Kennedy's legislation. In 1965, riding on this wave of enthusiasm, Congress added funding for staffing grants to the CMHC legislation. In the early 1960s, training in psychiatry included extremely little in the way of social science of "community" psychiatry since the medicalization of treatment and theory had long since become dominant in psychiatry. The public health rhetoric, sounding much like a social science challenge to this medicalization, actually stressed medicalized treatments expanded into local clinic settings. Nonetheless, public health psychiatry had won a major victory with CMHC legislation, and many expected radically different, "community" models of care to emerge from the ranks of psychiatry—the discipline now charged with control of a new, national network of centers. Center directors, by law, had to be psychiatrists, another sign that the movement was meant to expand the psychiatric market place.

The need to develop and staff centers with community oriented psychiatrists presented a problem to a discipline with few community oriented personnel. As Dr. Gerald Caplan, an academic community psychiatrist, wrote [16, p.69]:

> . . . to retain our leadership we must accept the legislators' offer to rise to the challenge of adjusting our professional theories and practices to the new situation which confronts us. . . . Perhaps we will be strengthened in overcoming the inevitable obstacles by the realization that we have no reasonable alternative.

Clearly, psychiatry had to unite under the banner of community care or be overshadowed by the large numbers of non-psychiatric therapists flooding into the market as the number of available positions grew. Indeed psychologists, clinical social workers, psychiatric nurses, even clinical sociologists were beginning to define their own pieces of the treatment market. One reflection of the growing turf rivalries was the fight over the label "social psychology" [24, p. 68]. Psychiatrists, argued that psychologists had too little control over the clinical certification of social psychologists to grant them licenses to practice. It was felt that the fact that sociologists also used the term "social psychologist" muddied the practice waters for the public and so the American

Psychological Association asked the American Sociological Association to forbid its members from using the term social psychologists for sociologists. The request was denied. This was just one incident of the increasing interprofessional and inter-occupational tensions which intensified as the market expanded.

REGULATIONS AND AMENDMENTS

The first regulations specifying details of centers were issued in 1964. They included the requirements for provision of five basic services: in-patient care, out-patient care, emergency care, partial hospitalization, and consultation and education. Of the five, the first four were clearly related to individualized treatments, and only consultation and education seemed to be a radical departure. As will be shown later, even this service primarily implied an extension of the psychiatric domain to non-hospital settings such as schools and prisons.

Centers were mandated to be geographically responsible to catchment areas, areas defined to include between 75,000 and 200,000 persons. The regulations also required coordination among services, and coordination of information, staff, and clients.

States were mandated to specify target groups of especially needy potential clients, and to include these in their state mental health plans, along with suggested actions for meeting their needs. State planning was to target the existence of low income areas, chronic unemployed, substandard housing, alcoholism, drug abuse, crime and delinquency, as well as the special needs of the mentally handicapped, the aged and children [25]. The strategy of targeting special needs groups, and basing services on rational planning for geographic areas were principles adopted from public health.

Despite the lack of firm evidence that centers were influencing the continuing discharge of chronic patients from state hospitals, in 1965 Dr. Felix wrote [26, p. xxi]:

> I believe more firmly now than when I first made the statement a few years ago (during the original CMHC legislative hearings) that within two decades the public mental hospital as we know it will no longer exist because there will be no need for it. The community mental health center, if possible, tied into hospital facilities in the community, the family physician and the psychiatric specialist will be able to manage in the community all but the most complicated and difficult psychiatric cases.

Perhaps part of this optimism came from the fact that Dr. Felix, in the years since the establishment of the Joint Commission on Mental Health and Illness in 1955, had seen NIMH's budget go from about 18 million to over 300 million. As others had documented the Community Mental Health legislation meant NIMH had now expanded into the world of big business [27]. It was now funding large-scale direct services and programs in many areas of the social sciences. Dr. Felix's public health vision was now the foundation for public mental health policy.

By 1967, the CMHC construction grants were extended for three more years and staffing grants for two years. During the period from 1965 until 1969, 75 percent of the allotted funds for the program were actually authorized, amounting to approximately 195 million dollars [28].

Also, in 1967, new regulations were issued by HEW governing CMHC staffing and construction. As the Joint Information Service [29] (a service of the American Psychiatric Association and the National Association for Mental Health) reported after the new regulations were issued in March of 1967, NIMH had only four months left in the fiscal year to process applications and allot that year's staffing money. A wide variety of services were being funded with little scrutiny, and little systematic evaluation of results. In that one year, out of $19.5 million allotted, NIMH managed to spend $15 million [29, pp. 8-9].

Clearly, the CMHC movement was a major vehicle for extending the monopoly dominated, mental health service market at State expense. In doing so it was fulfilling the State functions of heightened accumulation and legitimation. Accumulation came in the form of a greatly expanded privatized market underwritten at public expense. Legitimation came in the form of mandating psychiatric control and greatly expanded mental illness treatment episodes. Although Kennedy died before funding of the program truly began, Johnson was able to use it as one part of his Great Society initiative aimed at controlling urban black unrest and carrying out what Piven and Cloward aptly called, *Regulating the Poor* [30]. As those authors documented, the modernization of agriculture in the South during the preceding decade disproportionately affected the black population, and, in important respects, created the conditions underlying the rise of black power movements in the 1950s and 1960s. Blacks began acquiring political power through waves of civil rights demonstrations and massive voter registration drives. Part of the civil rights movement's strategy was to arouse the power of local and state governments which opposed equal rights. Social control was often enforced through the brutal use of political and military power, a reaction which made good material for national television news coverage. The federal government, meanwhile, often sought to intervene in the form of social investments rather than force. Massive health, welfare and urban development expenditures were used as an alternative form of reaction and control. Kennedy's political support, after all, depended on the black vote in industrial areas, and Johnson later built on this base by promises of more aid and reform.

In the early 1960s, the CMHC program was one of many such forms of social investment targeted chiefly at urban areas, areas torn apart by racial unrest. Money flowed to youth development programs, community development programs, and mental health programs, among others. These monies were meant not only to help aid the poor and minority communities, but were seen as what Piven and Cloward called "program patronage" in return for black votes. Neighborhood residents were brought into storefront offices to serve local clientele with federal spoils. As they wrote [30, p. 261]:

> It made little difference whether the funds were appropriated under delinquency-prevention, mental health, antipoverty, or model-cities legislation: in the streets of the ghettoes, many aspects of the programs looked very much alike.

In this sense, the CMHC monies were federal social investments which reaped privatized profits for the monopoly sector.

PHASE II: CONTINUED MARKET EXPANSION AND WIDENED UNREST

By the late 1960s, urban unrest had diversified and spread. Civil rights activity had merged with other struggles including anti-war protests, counter-culture movements, feminist activity, and national liberation movements worldwide. These recurring waves of political activism were heightened by the continuing War in Vietnam. Repressive actions taken to quell anti-war protests only served to increase unrest throughout the nation. Such protests, along with the civil rights movement, were beginning to take on an international flavor. An increasing number of wars of liberation were flaring in Third World countries, and strikes and civil disturbances were occurring with increasing frequency in industrialized nations. The rise of communist movements in Italy, the revolution in Portugal, and the massive general strike in France, all in the late 1960s, reflected a generalized rise of political tension and sense of economic crisis in the capitalist world.

This was the new political and economic situation within which the CMHC movement flourished in the late 1960s. By 1969, inflation was rising and recession loomed in the United States. Continued federal support for the CMHC movement was the focus for mounting criticism. The initial enthusiasm over Kennedy's bold new approach to mental illness treatment was now blunted with pragmatic economic questions. At the same time, a list of woes was being recited by community mental health center directors who were trying to find alternative, "community" funding as federal monies dried up.

Movement critics began loudly charging that the spread of the CMHC movement was a blatant attempt at more State social control. Kenneth Kenniston [31], for example, described "How Community Mental Health Stamped Out the Riots (1968-1978)." Dr. Kenniston, tongue in cheek, reported on a "dream" he had, in which he saw Secretary for International Mental Health, General Westmoreland (sic. actually a key figure in the Vietnam War) who was Secretary for Internal Mental Health, and General Wald respond to "inner-city violence, alienation, and antisocial behavior." Their response was to expand community mental health care from 2800 centers to more than 5000, to define catchment areas to 'target groups,' and to include the idea of 'total therapy'—i.e. preventing socially disruptive objectivist issues like black power, civil rights, or improvement in living conditions through crisis intervention which was supplemented by 'prolonged aftercare.' The early ideals spoken of by the initiators of the CMHC movement had obviously been translated into the language of State social control.

Many authors took turns clashing over the proper conceptualization of social organization and community change, over the evolving division of labor among workers in the mental health services market, and over the organizational structures for CMHCs. For example, the *Handbook of Community Mental Health Practice: The San Mateo Experience*, published in 1969 [32] listed the following problems with the CMHC programs: inadequate conceptualization of the mission; lack of comprehensiveness; failure to provide complete services for a catchment area; absence of services to children, to old people; various interpretations of continuity of care; the changing of therapists when patients went from one service to another; role blurring between professionals, a tendency for minimal roles to be filled by the psychiatrists who principally served the medication patients; the failure to utilize general practitioners; the difficulty in identifying short-term and long-term patients at admission; the almost complete absence of day hospitals and partial hospitalization; deficient emergency care without personnel around the clock; poor understanding of consultation; the expressed need for more training in community health; the absence of relationships with state hospitals and the absence of evaluation and effectiveness measures of programs [32, p. x].

Many of these problems could be traced to the clash between the promise of innovation which had been the hallmark of the movement and the reality of traditional psychiatric care delivered in CMHCs. Social problems were not defined as "treatable" within this psychiatric tradition. Public health enthusiasm had not reached far into psychiatric training, and when it had, it offered few clear directions for action. CMHCs were having a hard time hiring psychiatric staff; salaries were relatively low; and the jobs offered seemed to be less than satisfactory, especially if psychiatrists were being asked to address social ills about which they knew little.

By the mid 1970s it was clear that demand for psychiatrists to work in CMHCs was growing faster than the supply. Lehman and Lehman analyzed various incentive structures to attract psychiatrists to community mental health work [33]. Their conclusions included the findings that while such normative factors as religion and political orientation did help predict which psychiatrists were willing to work in CMHCs, the most powerful predictor of choosing community work was the potential income it offered to psychiatrists. It was true that Protestant psychiatrists were more likely than Catholic or Jewish psychiatrists to undertake community mental health work, and that psychiatrists who were political leftist were more likely to work in CMHCs. Nonetheless, it seemed that the potential for high income was not a hallmark of community work and psychiatrists were hard to come by. Another issue was the potential for role discrepancy for medically trained personnel, especially nurses and psychiatrists, who worked in setting which many thought would move away from traditional, individualistic and organic definitions of mental disorder to innovative social orientations. Unlike what the innovators might have expected, role discrepancy was actually highest for social workers, psychologists, and paraprofessionals working in CMHCs who expected nontraditional orientations on the part of staff and administration but did not find it. Medically oriented staff nurses and psychiatrists, found the traditionality of most CMHCs to be exactly what they had been trained to expect.

The CMHC movement had not only engendered tremendous expansion of the service market for psychiatry, but also for social scientists who saw in the movement the potential for exploring a wide range of social and medical ills. The diversity of such approaches was documented, for example, by Duhl and Leopold who wrote about the collaboration of a young resident physician and an anthropologist who sought funds for a CMHC [19]. In an unusually frank and moving account of behind-the-scenes maneuvering, these authors recounted how local politics and interprofessional rivalries killed the funding possibilities.

The movement by this time had set one psychiatric faction off against another, i.e. public health psychiatry against other schools of psychiatry. It had also divided federal interests. Despite these clashes, the movement was continuing to fulfill the basic State functions cited earlier, those of accumulation for the privatized psychiatric market and legitimation for middle-class values. The activism of the late 1960s not only tested the coercive might of the State, but also the ideological control exercised by professionals who profited from the market conditions. Counter-culture groups, hippies, communal groups, feminists, black power activists and others rejected traditional cultural assumptions as to family, sex roles, religion and morality. All of these were frequently pictured as threats to the dominant class values. Cultural control seemed to be breaking; free love, drugs and nontraditional dress seemed to be effectively undercutting control of legitimate authority figures. Organizers were teaching the powerless how to gain a voice [34]. Economic pressures of the fiscal crisis, manifest in the late 1960s, also brought with them increasing stress on broad sectors of the population. Physical and psychiatric symptomatology paralleled swings in the economy [35, p. 606]. The promise of relief from symptomatology which was offered through the provision of mental and physical health care provided an increasingly potent means of social control. It fed into the spread of an ideology of individualized distress and individualized relief through treatment.

One indirect indicator of the use of health and mental health care as individualized control came in the form of the increase in the use of prescription drugs by the general population. For many, drugs seemed to provide a convenient and effective way to block out social stress. Prescription drug use increased markedly in the 1960s. From 1961 until 1972, there was an increase of 100 percent or more in manufacturers' sales of most major categories of drugs, including the three largest types, i.e., central nervous system drugs, anti-infectives, and the category which included contraceptives [36]. The use of Valium and Librium for a wide variety of social stresses became extremely widespread. Valium, introduced in 1963, became the most frequently prescribed drug in the United States by 1972. "Three billion tablets of Valium and one billion tablets of Librium were sold in the United States in 1974, enough for one week of drug therapy for every person in the United States" [36, p. 38].

Mental health care services were provided with a tremendous federal investment, expanding service markets in the form of the community mental health centers, but this was only part of the total health care expenditure. With the advent of Medicare and Medicaid, socialized costs of social consumption in health rose dramatically. The federal expenditures in health rose from slightly over 2,102 millions of dollars in 1960 to over 15,000 millions of dollars in 1971. The percent of total health expenditures accounted for by the federal sector went from 9.2 percent of the total in 1960, to 22.9 percent in 1971. By comparison, in the preceding five years, it had gone from a high of 10.4 percent in 1955 down to 9.2 percent in 1960 [21, p. 387].

For mental health care in particular, rates of care episodes rose dramatically from 1028 per 100,000 population in 1955; to 1376 per 100,000 in 1965; to 1977 per 100,000 in 1971. In terms of community mental health centers, their share of the market had gone from 0 percent in the mid 1960s to 15 percent by 1971, accounting for over 600,000 care episodes in 1971 [37, p. 93].

As CMHCs became an institutionalized element of care, more emphasis was placed on the importance of third party reimbursement. This was increasingly so as CMHC federal funding was to be "stepped down" over a period of years. CMHC's history cannot be separated from the history of Medicaid, Medicare, and Supplemental Security Income (SSI) legislation. An analysis of this interconnectedness comes in Levine's 1981 work *The History and Politics of Community Mental Health* [38]. Levine documented how such reimbursement programs helped shift significant numbers of elderly and disabled patients from state hospitals to alternative sites of care, often nursing homes or single room occupancy (SROs) dwellings — frequently with little care or oversight. The author pointed up the lack of coordination between funding programs and between state hospitals and community settings. As Levine wrote [38, p. 77]:

Programs and policies that interacted with mental health programs and shaped them developed without any apparent consideration for the effect of one piece of legislation on another, and without regard for the tendencies of bureaucracies to pursue their own ends, almost independently of legislative intent or authorization.

It is understandable within this context that legal issues such as criteria for commitment, sites of treatment, rights to treatment, and patient's rights emerged as central social and political issues. Along with the burgeoning of legal cases came an increasing dialogue between mental health professionals, often psychiatrists, and the legal profession over the role of each in the lives of those formally defined as mentally ill. Levine also addressed this aspect of the history, tracing how attempts at legal redress for patients often ended in little substantive change in the fragmented care system [38].

Along with the great increase in federal funding, and the tremendous market expansion, came great complexity and fragmentation in the political and economic interests within the CMHC movement. The rather small coalition of psychiatrists and federal politicians who had initiated the movement in the earlier part of the decade, were now joined by a huge number of warring special interests by late in the decade. In a study by the Rand Corporation, and cited in a 1972 article by Bertram Brown, (Director of NIMH in the late 1960s and early 1970s) and James W. Stockdill, "The Politics of Mental Health," [39] the mental health power structure was now crowded with suppliers, allies, beneficiaries, rivals and others. NIMH now sat in the middle of rival political powers, represented by Congress and HEW, academic and research interests and numerous voluntary associations and professional groups. As those authors forthrightly stated [39, p. 682]:

With the development of community mental health programs more was required than merely clinical science and technology and facilities planning and administration.

Consideration by the mental health professional now had to be given not only to the patient's social setting but also to the political setting in which the programs themselves were developing and operating. 'The success of a mental health program is no longer simply a function of clinical skills of the program staff; the success of the program is equally dependent on skills in coping with, adapting to, and sometimes even changing the local political, social and economic environment.'

The increasingly complex division of labor was another aspect of the market expansion which moved it beyond control of the original coalition of CMHC leaders. Despite their early vision of the movement as thoroughly under the control of psychiatry, and of centers being rather traditional "doctors' workshops" such as were the community hospitals, by 1972 CMHCs were much more heavily dependent on non-psychiatric staff than on psychiatrists. Mental health workers, often local persons with less than a B. A. degree, accounted for 50 percent of the full-time equivalent patient care positions in centers by 1972, and psychiatrists and other M. D.s accounted jointly for slightly over 7 percent of those positions [37, p. 19]. By 1970, psychiatric input into the centers had peaked, and it headed down throughout the following decade [40]. Off setting this decline was the input by psychologists, social workers and registered nurses [37]. Middle-level and upper-level therapeutic personnel had found in the CMHC movement a bonanza for their employment markets. These persons used the movement to gain footholds in the therapeutic marketplace while being employed as State workers. Corporate interests also continued to benefit since their drugs and treatment markets expanded along with increased care episodes.

Class, sex and race distinctions among levels and types of CMHC personnel remained pronounced. Psychiatrists were, by and large, well-paid white males. Social workers and nurses were paid considerably less, and were usually women, white or minority. Navarro presented an analysis of sex and income differences for the health marketplace as a whole [41]. He noted that in 1970, the top strata of workers consisted of physicians and administrators who earned a median income of $40,000 a year. The middle strata of therapists and nurses earned a median income of $6,000 a year. On the bottom were the largest numbers of workers, overwhelmingly women, earning a median income of $4,000 a year. For CMHCs, this lowest strata accounted for over one-third of the total-full time equivalent staff by 1970 [37, p. 484].

In O'Connor's terms, by the late 1960s, the State (in this case, largely the federal government) had socialized the costs of the mental illness treatment market, but the majority of profits were fed back to the monopoly sector which included drug and related industries, and high paid administrators and psychiatrists [10]. By expanding the marketplace, however, the division of labor had also been increased when huge numbers of competitive sector workers had been hired by the State to expand the lower ranks of the labor pool. By 1969-1970, the federal government began to worry increasingly about inflation and recession and needed to look toward the monopoly sector to support its own infrastructural costs [10]. The State was compelled to increase efficiency in the State sector, including federal programs, and to stabilize market expansion [10, p. 51]. The continuing increase in social investment, as compared to the investment of private capital, in market expansion for the monopoly sector, was reaching a critical turning point [10, p. 24]. At the same time, the 1969 recession was hitting just when dependency on federal support programs, such as welfare, was booming. One reason these programs had expanded so quickly was that they expanded private markets and provided State social control during years of general social unrest [30, p. 341]. The change from expansion of federal expenditure, including CMHC's, to consolidation and rationalization of expenditures amounted to a change from regulating civil disorder to regulating the increased labor market [30, p. 342]. By 1972, the impact of this change was clearly visible in the CMHC program.

Despite all the attention given to the move to deinstitutionalize in the United States, Northern Europeans had actually begun the process several decades earlier. Data suggest that the move away from long-term in-patient stays and the rise of shorter in-patient stays, open wards, along with the use of groups homes and alternative living arrangements can be dated from the 1940s—at least a half decade before the introduction of chlorpromazine. Warner, who analyzed data from ten Western nations, made a strong case that this shift not only served to save the additional dollars it would have cost governments to maintain and expand public institutional care, i.e. indoor relief, but closely paralleled the need for labor [42]. In times of full employment in Postwar Europe, the demand for labor "stimulated truly rehabilitative forms of social therapy, designed to bring marginally functional psychiatric patients into the labor force . . ." [42, p. 25].

In times of growing unemployment, the association between public mental hospital beds and the employment rate weakened according to Warner's analysis. Seemingly factors other than the need for labor became increasingly important in determining state policy [42, p. 27]. Such was the case by the early 1970s in the United States.

PHASE III: ECONOMIC AND POLITICAL CONSOLIDATION

By 1972, the by-word of the CMHC movement had become accountability. In an effort to cap the flow of federal funds, the Nixon administration looked toward a variety of measures from rationalizing expenditures, including the mandating of evaluation research on programs, to outright impoundment of authorized funds. U.S. Senate hearings in 1973 reported that the percent of authorized funds for CMHC's which were allocated dropped from 100 percent in 1965 and 1966, to 51 percent in 1970, and down to 17 percent in 1972. In actual dollars, this meant a drop from the 1965 level of spending of $35,000,000, to a 1972 level of $15,000,000 [28, p. 5]. Reflected in this drop was a deep division within branches of the federal government, legislative versus executive, over the CMHC program. By 1972, Brown and Stockdill could write in their political analysis of the situation [39, p. 672]:

> ... there is general agreement that much of the credit of mental health's sound national legislative base of the 1960s can be attributed to the ear of legislators Fogarty and Hill. However, their era is over.

Their era had ended in the crush of new interests into the mental health services arena in the 1960s, and in the fiscal crisis of the late 1960s. Between 1955 and 1975, the mental health care episodes in in-patient and out-patient facilities had increased fivefold. The pattern of care had gone from overwhelmingly in-patient, 77 percent in the mid 1950s, to overwhelmingly out-patient, 72 percent by the 1970s [37, p. 330]. Nixon now sought to dismantle the Kennedy-Johnson programs. Dr. Yolles resigned as director of NIMH in opposition to Nixon's stand, and in his place Dr. Bernard Brown, a consummate politician and believer in program rationalization, was appointed.

One of the first federal moves toward rationalization came in 1971. In that year the Comptroller General of the United States issued a report to Congress, "The Community Mental Health Centers Program—Improvement Needed in Management" [43]. The report reviewed the processes and outcomes of CMHC grants including by 1970, $230,000,000 in grants for construction and $217,000,000 in staffing grants. The authors documented how some states had used areas larger than the designated catchment areas for planning, how no NIMH national goals on numbers of centers had been set, how some construction grants seemed to have been larger than warranted (for example, some monies had gone to support areas shared between centers and hospitals), how insufficient information on evaluation of proposed size of in-patient facilities was available, how no criteria on in-patient services in relationship to area needs was available, how a need existed for a realistic appraisal of an applicant's ability to obtain sufficient non-federal funds for a center's operation and for monitoring the center's financial status after funds were awarded, and how staffing grant money was being used for unauthorized or questionable purposes at several centers [43, p. 2]. In the course of their work, these investigators had found evidence of considerable discrepancy between funding guidelines and actual spending. For example, although centers were supposed to be ranked and funded by "need," as specified in state plans, California and Florida had been funding centers with little regard to prioritization.

This report, and others from the executive branch, provided the anti-CMHC forces with the data they sought. Ironically, by now, critics included both fiscal conservatives and liberals. The latter charged that the programs were really attempts at State social control. As described by Bloom [44, p. 50]:

> On June 18, 1973, just before the expiration date of the twice extended Community Mental Health Centers Act, Congress enacted the Health Program Extension Act of 1973 (Public Law 93-45), which authorized funds for a one-year extension of a large number of federally-supported health programs, including the community mental health centers program. Prior to this, extreme differences of opinion, both within Congress and between Congress and the executive branch of government, that had existed since the start of the Nixon era had broken through the surface, as the White House made it known that it strongly opposed the continued funding of the community mental health center and other programs.

The differences cited by Bloom involved several factions: 1) the CMHC old guard who were still supporting the original intent of market expansion and humanized care in local community centers; 2) the liberals who supported expansion of social programs in general, but who questioned social control motives; and 3) the fiscal conservatives who wanted to cap federal spending. This last group was led by the executive branch under Nixon. In response to Nixon's impoundment of CMHC monies, NIMH asked congress to clarify the purposes of the centers, their model of care (medical or social), the continued role of federal funding, the limits of the catchment concept, the advisability of mandated services for all centers, and the concept of accessibility [44, p. 52]. This tactic gave the Congressional factions additional time to compromise, and it also gave the chief sponsors of the Act, along with NIMH, time to consolidate their positions.

In 1974, the Congress again grappled with the CMHC legislation, but avoided direct answers to NIMH's questions. This time it was the administration of President Ford, not of President Nixon, which responded to the CMHC Act with a veto of the bill. The two year extension of funding for CMHC's was now tied in Congress to increased mandatory services including services for the elderly, children, consultation to courts and to other agencies, follow-up care, and halfway houses [44, p. 53].

The special interest groups representing these target groups or services had achieved success in their lobbying efforts. In addition to providing these newly mandated special services, CMHC's were to add assurances of quality of care, and integration of old services with new. The fiscal conservatives had won this latter addition as a concession to their concerns about control over services. The CMHC legislation was, however, tied to a large package of other social programs, programs left over from the Johnson Great Society years. The fiscal conservatives persuaded Ford to veto the package. Congress recessed before it could override the veto.

Liberals, meantime, had consolidated their own attacks on the program. In the same year as the conservative battles over funding and the Ford veto occurred, Ralph Nader's organization published its own hard criticism of CMHC's, *The Madness Establishment*, by Chu and Trotter [4]. This attack represented a change from the radical critique of the late 1960s, a critique often emanating from radical mass movements. The new language of liberal criticism was the language of the middle-class consumer movement, a liberal rationalistic response to what was seen as unresponsiveness in government and business to middle-class needs and interests.

The Madness Establishment [4], was a wide ranging analysis of CMHC management and planning failures. The authors cited, among other issues, the lack of clear relationships between centers, poor services for the disadvantaged, a lack of coordination and planning, little evaluation and no accountability for centers to Congress or to consumers. Overall, the authors criticized the CMHC movement for what they saw as its ill defined and hasty implementation. They charged that it was a piece of legislation dependent on federal franchise granted to elite medical/psychiatric interests and used by the elites to monopolize care.

Similar conclusions were reached by Ellison et al. who wrote that the Federal Guidelines for CMHC were so inflexible and ambiguous that "nearly any function, new or old, can be carried out in the name of community mental health" [45, p. 180]. Such functions could include an entirely new structure, part of an existing system; couples, individuals or agencies hired to carry out programs; grants awarded to groups of incorporated citizens or institutions; part of teaching hospitals and training programs; personnel hired full or part-time; and center staff trained by professional or community people. Federal monies were going to pay for all of these and any combination.

By 1976, the federal outlays for "improving" the organization and delivery of health services had mushroomed as part of the account-ability trend. They had grown from $117,000,000 in 1969 to $424,000,000 in 1976. [46, p. 60]. CMHC funding, and other mental health monies targeted at organizational improvement, had grown from $16,000,000 in 1969 to $112,000,000 in 1976 [46].

The CMHC legislation of mid-decade reflected this move to market consolidation. The 1975 extension of the Act provided for program planning, construction and staffing; it also emphasized consultation and education and comprehensive services such as additions to existing services in centers which were having staffing grants terminated. Beyond this, the legislation mandated services to targeted special interest groups such as children and the elderly, and it required diag-nostic, treatment, liaison and follow-up care. Screening for treatment, and halfway houses were to be supported. Alcohol and drug prevention were also mandated. The authors of the bill insisted on improving collaboration among mental health agencies, and on improving the provision of services to culturally and economically distinct groups who had previously been "under-served." The legislation also called for citizen participation and continuous quality assurance, as well as con-fidentiality for patient information [44, p. 55]. In all, twelve mandated services had found their way into the CMHC Act, a multiplicity of mandated services which tested the administrative skills of even large, university-based centers, let alone store front clinics.

These new legislative mandates again reflected the struggle within the federal government between CMHC true believers in Con-gress and NIMH, liberal reformers, and fiscal conservatives. They also reflected the power of numerous special interest lobbies, lobbies for agencies serving children, the elderly, drug addicts, and others. The Great Society had brought not only urban blacks into political par-ticipation through social investment, but had helped support the growth of vast numbers of services, staffed by competitive and related sector personnel—personnel who occupied a structural position be-tween monopoly interests and competitive sector workers. If funding was to be rationalized or cut, these persons all were facing the potential of seeing their salaries "rationalized" away. These interests were especially vocal in the fight not to be pushed out of the market or left out of the legislation when infrastructural costs were transferred to the private sector.

With the coming of the Carter administration, the CMHC movement was brought into its final years. A new director of NIMH was appointed by Carter, and a new President's Commission on Mental Health was appointed to study national mental health needs and services. Mrs. Rosalyn Carter was appointed Honorary Chairperson of the Commission, and her interest in mental illness services was an important element in this effort.

After a year of study, Presidential Task Force Panels presented their reports and recommendations to the President. The resultant *Report to the President,* and the three volume Task Panel Reports of the President's Commission on Mental Health represented a new effort at forming a federal coalition to support legislation, just as had the Joint Commission in its report two decades earlier. The elite psychiatric and corporate interests involved in the 1955 work had now been replaced or overshadowed by a myriad of special interests crowding the treatment market. The strong voices of these interests could be heard in the language of Task Panels, and they were often legitimated by CMHC evaluation research undertaken in the mid 1970s.

The outcome of the Commission's work was a new piece of federal legislation, the Mental Health Systems Act, replacing the earlier CMHC Act with a newly conceptualized approach to services. Rather than mandating twelve services in one center, the Systems Act funded phased-in "systems" of services. Rather than providing direct federal funding, the Systems Act called for turning monies back to states for distribution through individual state departments of mental health. Local and state political organizations, locked out of funding in the Great Society era, now re-emerged as winners in the struggle for control. The cries of the fiscal conservatives for less government intervention had been translated into a "New Federalism," a new reliance on local political control and the private sector.

By the end of the decade of the 1970s, proposed realignments were underway. With the coming of the 1980s, and the Reagan Administration, not only the CMHC Act, but the Mental Health Systems Act was in danger of total defunding. In fact, it was lumped into block grants with numerous other social programs and was eventually forgotten in the rush to save whatever federal monies could be saved for such programs. The era of federal investment in mental illness care had ended, at least as far as the initial vision of community mental health centers. As authors in the early 1980s predicted, much of the policy attention regarding mental health services in the 1980s returned to the states and to the role of state hospitals in caring for the chronically mentally ill. (A fuller discussion of the 1980s is set forth in Chapter 7—Aftermath.)

The CMHC movement had been just one part of what O'Connor referred to as the social industrial complex—joint ventures between industry and the State to provide the conditions for privatized, monopoly profits by expanding the market infrastructure [10]. The withdrawal of federal support created the conditions for factionalism among interests who battled for their share of the market. The withdrawal of federal support also tested the divided loyalties represented within the State, i.e. the Congress, NIMH, and the federal branch. Not only had State control brought large numbers of personnel into the treatment service market, but it had provided a potential basis or organization among the market's labor pool. As O'Connor suggested [10, p. 241]:

> What are the qualitative aspects of labor struggle within the state sector, particularly struggles engaged in by service workers— teachers, social and welfare workers, probation personnel, city planners, employees in recreation, and so forth? On the one hand, the education of service workers consists largely of technical scientific training. They are taught the rudiments of scientific method, the history of their "profession," their obligations as public servants, and so on. In the course of their education and work experience service workers learn that society consists of a system of social relations that can be modified or totally transformed. On the other hand, the fusion of economic base and political superstructure and the fiscal crisis have led to the 'rationalization' of state jobs, the introduction of efficiency criteria, the waning of professional standards, and in general the transplantation of capitalist norms from direct production in the private economy to the state administration.

This could just as well have been a summing up of the CMHC story.

Much of the CMHC labor pool was left without an organized structure or shared consciousness. Since the CMHC movement had not been a mass-based movement, it lacked even a partially unified, socially defined constituency beyond the numerous interests involved in the treatment market. The original leaders, elite psychiatrists and federal administrators, had long since been replaced on the federal scene by factionated special interests. The changed market structure and political climate left little hope for continued market expansion. Contradictions between State interests over accumulation and legitimation, and individual state interests over local markets and local political control, dealt the final death blow to the movement.

SUMMARY

Had the CMHC movement been a mass-based movement at the grass roots level, its history might well have been very different. It might have sprung from charismatic leadership which was able to generate an ideology of innovative care for an audience of true believers. It might have started from a constituency ready to be catalyzed first by reformist goals and later held together by a growing bureaucratic organization. In actuality, the CMHC movement was largely a product of a small number of mental health reformers in coalition with federal legislators and bureaucrats. The movement, set in motion by these leaders, served the interests of expanding the private mental illness market at public expense. It also served as a means for State legitimation and control during a historical period of turmoil. As the economic and political context of the movement changed, the latent function of the movement changed to that of a battle among middle-level service personnel over their share of the market. As the fiscal crisis of the State heightened, federal political support began to be withdrawn, intensifying such struggles.

One of the most potent instruments for catalyzing and sustaining federal and psychiatric support for the CMHC movement was the professional literature produced by those associated with the movement. In the following pages, the struggles on the political and economic front will be traced through the pages of this literature. The ebb and flow of various schools of theory will be shown to parallel the political and economic struggles described in this chapter.

REFERENCES

1. L. Bellak, Community Psychiatry: The Third Psychiatric Revolution, in *Handbook of Community Psychiatry and Community Mental Health*, L. Bellak (ed.), Grune and Stratton, New York, 1963.
2. B. L. Bloom, The Domain of 'Community Psychology,' *Journal of Community Psychology, 1*:1, pp. 8-11, 1973.

3. P. Reiff, Mental Health Manpower and Institutional Change, *American Psychologist, 21*, pp. 540-548, 1966.
4. F. D. Chu and S. Trotter, *The Madness Establishment*, Grossman Publishers, New York, 1974.
5. A. T. Scull, *Decarceration: Community Treatment and The Deviant— A Radical View*, Prentice-Hall, Inc., Englewood Cliffs, New Jersey, 1977.
6. P. Brown, *The Transfer of Care: Psychiatric De-institutionalization and Its Aftermath*, Routledge & Kegan Paul, Boston, 1985.
7. H. J. Brenner, *Mental Illness and the Economy*, Harvard University Press, Cambridge, Massachusetts, 1973.
8. R. Warner, Deinstitutionalization: How Did We Get Where We Are?, *Journal of Social Issues, 45*, pp. 17-30, 1989.
9. E. Mandel, *Late Capitalism*, Verso, London, 1975.
10. J. O'Connor, *The Fiscal Crisis of the State*, St. Martin's Press, New York, 1973.
11. R. H. Elling, The Fiscal Crisis of the State and State Financing of Health Care—Toward a Conceptual and Action Statement for Improved Public Support of Medicine and Health Care, *Social Science and Medicine, 15c*, pp. 207-217, 1981.
12. B. Bloom, *Changing Patterns of Psychiatric Care*, Brooks/Cole Publishers, Monterey, California, 1977.
13. H. A. Foley and S. Sharfstein, *Who Cares for the Mentally Ill?*, American Psychiatric Press, Washington, D.C., 1983.
14. P. Conrad and J. W. Schneider, *Deviance and Medicalization: From Badness to Sickness*, The C. V. Mosby Company, St. Louis, 1980.
15. R. Brown, *Rockefeller Medicine Men: Medicine and Capitalism in America*, University of California Press, Berkeley, 1979.
16. D. F. Musto, Whatever Happened to Community Mental Health?, *The Public Interest, 39*, pp. 53-78, 1975.
17. R. H. Connery, C. H. Backstrom, J. R. Friedman, R. H. Marden, P. Meekison, D. R. Deener, M. Kroll, C. McCleskey, and J. A. Morgan, Jr., *Politics of Mental Health: Organizing Community Mental Health in Metropolitan Areas*, Columbia Press, New York, 1968.
18 A. M. Rossi, Some Pre-World War II Antecedents of Community Mental Health Theory and Practice, *Mental Hygiene, 46*, pp. 78-94, 1962.
19. L. J. Duhl and R. L. Leopold (eds.), *Mental Health and Urban Society*, Jossey-Bass, San Francisco, 1969.
20. H. A. Foley and S. Sharfstein, *Madness and Government: Who Cares for the Mentally Ill?*, American Psychiatric Association, Washington, D.C., 1983.
21. U.S. Department of H.E.W./H.H.S., *Health*, U.S. Department of H.E.W., Washington, D.C., 1978.
22. R. Fein, *Economies of Mental Illness*, Basic Books, New York, 1958.

23. J. F. Kennedy, *Message from the President of the United States Relative to Mental Illness and Mental Retardation*, 88th Congress, 1st Session, House Doc. 58, General Printing Office, Washington, D.C., 1963.
24. Goode, 1960 as quoted in M. Spector and J. I. Kitsuse, *Constructing Social Problems*, Aldine, New York, 1987.
25. R. Cohen, Neglected Legal Dilemmas in Community Psychiatry, in *Sociological Perspectives on Community Mental Health*, P. M. Roman and H. M. Rice, (eds.), P. A. Davis Co., Philadelphia, pp. 69-82, 1974.
26. R. L. Epps, R. H. Barnes, and T. S. McPartland, *A Community Concern: Experiences with Management of Major Mental Illness in the Community*, Charles C. Thomas, Springfield, Illinois, 1965.
27. F. D. Chu and S. Trotter, *The Madness Establishment*, Grossman Publishers, New York, 1974.
28. U.S. Senate, Health Subcommittee of the Committee on Labor and Public Welfare, *Community Mental Health Centers Act*, History of the Program and Current Problems and Issues, Government Printing Office, Washington, D.C., pp. 93-104, 1973.
29. Joint Information Service, *The Community Mental Health Center: An Interim Appraisal*, Joint Information Service, Washington, D.C., 1969.
30. F. F. Piven and R. A. Cloward, *Regulating the Poor: The Functions of Public Welfare*, Random House, New York, 1972.
31. K. Kenniston, How Community Mental Health Stamped Out the Riots (1968-1978), *Trans-action, 5:S*, pp. 21-29, 1968.
32. W. E. Barton, *Handbook of Community Mental Health Practice: The San Mateo Experience*, Human Sciences Press, New York, 1969.
33. E. W. Lehman and E. Lehman, Psychiatrists and Community Mental Health: Normative Versus Utilitarian Incentives, *Journal of Health and Social Behavior, 17:4*, pp. 364-375, 1976.
34. S. D. Alinsky, *Rules for Radicals*, Random House, New York, 1971.
35. H. Brenner, Economic Changes and Heart Disease Morality, *American Journal of Public Health, 65*, 1971.
36. I. Waldron, Increased Prescribing of Valium, Librium, and Other Drugs—An Example of the Influence of Economic and Social Factors on the Practice of Medicine, *International Journal of Health Services, 7:1*, pp. 37-61, 1977.
37. President's Commission on Mental Health, *Report to the President and Task Panel Reports*, Government Printing Office, Washington, D.C., Vol. II, 1978.
38. M. Levine, *The History and Politics of Community Mental Health*, Oxford Press, New York, 1981.
39. B. M. Brown and J. W. Stockdill, The Politics of Mental Health, in *Handbook of Community Mental Health*, S. E. Golann and C. Eisdorfer (eds.), Appleton-Century-Crofts, New York, pp. 669-686, 1972.

40. R. Bass and L. D. Ozarin, Community Mental Health Center Program: What Is Past Is Prologue, Annual Meeting of the American Psychiatric Association, Toronto, Canada, 1977.
41. V. Navarro, *Medicine Under Capitalism*, Prodist, New York, 1976.
42. R. Warner, Deinstitutionalization: How Did We Get Where We Are?, *Journal of Social Issues, 45*:3, pp. 17-30, 1989.
43. Comptroller General of the United States, *The Community Mental Health Centers Program—Improvements Needed in Management*, Department of H.E.W., Washington, D.C., 1971.
44. Bernard L. Bloom, *Community Mental Health: A General Introduction*, Brooks/Cole Publishers, Co., Monterey, California, 1977.
45. D. L. Ellison, P. Rieker, and J. H. Marx, Organizational Adaptation to Community Mental Health: A Case Study, in *Sociological Perspectives on Community Mental Health*, P. Roman and H. Trice (eds.), F. A. Davis, Philadelphia, pp. 179-194, 1974.
46. M. S. Koleda, C. Burke, and J. S. Williams, *The Federal Health Dollar: 1969-1976*. The National Planning Association, Washington, D.C., 1977.

CHAPTER 5

Theory during Phase One when Consensus Dominates the Early Years, the Late 1950s to the Mid 1960s

How was the concept of community, an essentially sociological concept, applied in the literature of the CMHC movement during each of the three political economic phases? The answer to this seemingly straightforward question occupies most of the rest of this book. What will be shown in the next three chapters is that as the political economic needs of the movement altered, so too did the application of theory. These changes will be delineated by tracing the changing use of the concept community as it was applied as a consensual or conflictual concept.

Unfortunately, most scholarly reviews of theory in the movement's literature shed little light on how and why certain theoretical approaches were adopted. One systematic approach to the question was undertaken by Lounsbury et al. who reported on a content analysis of titles of articles which were published in the *Community Mental Health Journal* [1]. As those authors found, there had been a general decrease in the number of "think pieces" and a general increase in matters of administrative concern over the years 1965 to 1976. Such might be the case with the literature from any social movement as it evolved from innovation to an institutionalized part of society. A more interesting conclusion was that although emphasis on the expansion of services into the community and the administrative details of justifying such expansion had been discussed repeatedly, issues of defining community, of shifting control over care to the community, and of changing the community itself had been largely ignored. As was argued by those authors [1, p. 274]:

> Emphasis in the field has been on (a) practice in community settings; (b) indirect rather than direct services; (c) new strategies for meeting the mental health needs of large numbers of people; (d) rational planning and decision making; and (e) innovative uses of human resources. On the other hand attention in the field has not been extensively addressed to four other important concerns mentioned by Bloom (2): (a) the total community or total defined population rather on individual patients or small subgroups; (b) preventive activities; (c) community control and citizen participation in mental health delivery systems; and (d) identifying sources of psycho-social stress in the community. Other potentially important directions that are not actively pursued in the field are the creation of health-producing environments and mechanisms for enhancing the quality of life.

Although attention to issues of the community and delivery systems may not have been paramount in this journal, such issues were not ignored altogether. In fact, much of what was published about them was part of the literature of applied sociological theory.

Where such issues were discussed, they often reflected not only the professional socialization and ideological tilt of the author, but also the personal, applied experiences of the author in the CMHC movement. Some authors were clinicians and their words reflected an "insiders" view of the movement. Others were academics from a wide range of disciplines who were participant-observers which gave them more of an "outsiders" view. Still others were policy makers, planners, or general social commentators. The application of sociological theory also reflected each of these perspectives as the following discussion shows.

THEORY IN PHASE ONE

Community as Market and Community as Catchment Area

The literature of the early years of the CMHC movement did indeed reflect the tome and content of discovery, of testing, and of experimentation among medical psychiatric professionals. As have earlier noted, Dr. Felix, Director of NIMH and a key movement initiator, was totally committed to a public health model of care. Translated into policies, this meant the expansion of settings for psychiatric care, focusing care away from state hospitals, and a newly expanded federal role in mental health care. The talk of innovative primary prevention or community consultation was less easily framed into policy directives because they represented significant departures from the traditional medical model.

The central conceptual and ideological terms which both held these policies together and added the needed political underpinnings was "community." What wasn't stated, however, was that "the community" for doctors was quite certainly not the "community" of the politician or everyday citizen. In fact, when one looks at "the community" as discussed, for example, in the initial legislative hearings on the CMHC act, the doctors' community most often could be translated into the doctors' market area.

In the initial CMHC hearings, Dr. Francis Braceland, past president of the American Psychiatric Association and national figure in American psychiatry, was asked about the need to add staffing grants (a major sticking point of the legislation) to the construction monies. He replied [3, p. 57]:

> I feel it is extremely important, Senator Hill, because the community is going to have to be educated to this. . . . If we get the patients in there and get help—Federal help—in the staffing . . . then as it gets going the community will be able to move in, the local doctors will be able to move in and . . . there will be a change for private practice for service and the change for insurance to cover treatment in the centers. . . .

Here the community, whatever its composition, was seen as being closely identified with physicians and their markets. In fact, from this psychiatrist's viewpoint, the community melded into the image of the local doctors.

This being the case, it is not difficult to understand why four out of the five initially mandated services under the CMHC Act were clearly based on traditional models of care: inpatient, outpatient, emergency, and partial hospitalization. Only consultation and education were seen as innovative. What model were these based upon? One hint comes from the same initial hearings and the testimony of Dr. Nicholas Hobbs, speaking for the American Psychological Association [3, pp. 98-99]:

> The hope of the community mental health center, indeed the very cause of its emergence, as the promising new development in the mental health field, is a recognition that mental disorders are

more than, and in unique ways different from, most other illnesses or disabilities. They grow out of, are exacerbated by, and contribute to family and community disorganization. This position does not deny the existence or importance of genetic physiological or biochemical variables in the etiology of mental disturbance. It does emphasize that mental disorders are inexplicably bound up with child rearing practices, education, employment, recreation, health, religion—in sum, with the totality of family and community life.

This statement represents a rather conservative view of society; disorganization is one basis of personal pathology. Family and community disorganization can be very differently interpreted depending on whether they are spoken of within the context of priestly social structure or prophetic class struggle. The priestly view may emphasize traditional, white, middle-class ideals. The prophetic view may give equal standing to non-traditional units, for example, homosexual couples. Further, power relations within the family may be interpreted to reflect "normal" gender and status roles they may be seen to reflect exploitative norms from the larger society. These differing assumptions have far reaching consequences for the form and process of consultation, as will be discussed later in this chapter through the works of Gerald Caplan.

How were these definitions translated into legislative language for the CMHC Act? The Act read [4, p. 7]:

> The term "community mental health center" means a facility providing services for the prevention or diagnosis of mental illness, or care and treatment of mentally ill patients, or rehabilitation of such persons, which are provided principally for persons residing in a particular community or communities in or near which the facility is situated.

The regulations for Title II of the Act, Public Law 88-164, did little to clarify the meaning, adding only [5, p. 286]:

> Area means the geographic territory which includes one or more communities served or to be served by existing or proposed community mental health facilities, the delineation of which is based on such factors as population distribution, natural geographic boundaries, and transportation accessibility. . . . 'Community' means an area or that portion of an area served or to be served by a program providing at least the essential elements of comprehensive mental health services as specified . . .

Later in the regulations, area was translated into planning areas consisting of between 75,000 and 200,000 persons. "Catchment areas," a concept adopted from English planning literature, became the administrative term for community.

The relationship between these planning terms and "community" was rarely well-defined, and often disputed. For example, in 1969, the Joint Information Service, a group jointly sponsored by the American Psychiatric Association and NIMH, held a conference on the CMHC movement, and among the issues addressed was the usefulness of catchmenting.

The administrative director of one Center in Kansas, responding to the question of what community meant, stated [6, p. 40]:

> In our catchment area in Western Kansas, there are twenty-two counties. I can't think of anything except geography that makes these counties a community. It's just an arbitrary selection of counties.

The director of a Washington CMHC stated [6, p. 40]:

> Virtually every member agency of our center in Tacoma, Washington, has a different concept of 'community.' They certainly have differing concepts of 'catchment.' Some serve part or all of the city, some serve part or all of the county, some serve more than the county, and one serves a sizable portion of the state.
>
> My idea of community is related less to geography than to interlocking the inter-working relationships which create, for example, the "business community" and the "mental health service community." Such relationships don't have a lot to do with geography.

And the clinical director of another Center responded [6, p. 40]:

> In our area of North Dakota, which I lived for the past twenty years, the 'community' has fluctuated, as the result of trends in business, new roads, the movement of people in and out. Our catchment area for purposes of the community mental health center program is small compared to the total of people who for many years have come to our city for medical care from a very large radius.

This early transformation of community into catchment did cut legitimate boundaries for the marketing of CMHC services. These market areas were, in fact, franchises granted to the CMHC by the federal government. The catchment design was adopted throughout the nation despite misgivings on the part of some, such as the doctor who at the same Joint Information Service conference said, "The arrangement operates in restraint of competition and some of the franchises have gone to facilities that are not up to scratch" [6, p. 44].

Arguments over the catchment concept continued throughout the history of the movement. Both the theoretical transformation of community into geographic area and the practical fallout of this transformation attracted attention.

In 1972, Perlmutter and Silverman [7] published an article in a social work journal describing CMHC's as "structural anachronisms" largely because of the territorial administrative structure of many CMHC's based, in part, on the catchmenting concept.

One year later, in 1973, Huffine et al. published an analysis of the impact of catchmenting on the population served by a treatment unit at Johns Hopkins in Baltimore [8]. Their conclusion was that the catchmenting failed as a method of designing appropriate services for the needs of that community.

Despite such statements, the transformation of "community" into catchment areas did serve the need of the market. It allowed franchises, noncompetitive service units, to be established by local professional interests and to have them funded by the federal government. All of this occurred despite the fact that the catchment area ignored the dynamic aspects of ethnic, racial, and income characteristics of areas. This easy definition of community was the first and perhaps the most far reaching definition of community. It allowed easy identification of a community by planners and administrators within the CMHC movement, and it set the stage for the expansion of services. Unfortunately, it required only minimal knowledge of the social and cultural networks which linked people together. The definition and legitimation of the doctors' market area was quite like the definition of any business market area—it needed only to serve as a basic unit for estimating potential consumer demand in that area.

COMMUNITY AS SYSTEMS

Klein

What were authors in the early professional literature saying about the "community" from a theoretical point of view? Donald Klein, an important proponent of the public health model, wrote a 1965 article for *Community Mental Health Journal*, entitled "The Community and Mental Health: An Attempt at a Conceptual Framework" [9].

One could hardly ask for a clearer *consensual, priestly* overview of community than that presented by Klein, who seemed to take an eclectic approach by including long listings of "parts" of the overall system. He listed many characteristics of community including size, population density, location, resources, and topology (regional characteristics). He also suggested that one could look at the community through analysis of its structural characteristics, its authority, power and prestige structures, or communications within the community. His own approach was what he called a dynamic interplay of community forces seen as an "integrated field of forces," a "dynamic system" within which each segment is related to each other and exists in "equilibrium a balance of forces" [9, 10].

The key words of "integrated field" and "system" revealed that Klein was adopting a view of community as a system of mutually interacting subsystems in a state of equilibrium which tend toward self-maintenance. This is the basis of the priestly, consensual model outlined earlier. This concept of field or system (the two overlap in meaning, usually field implies a more fluid system with permeable boundaries than does system when used alone) is easily wedded to the administrative/planning use of catchmenting. Since the community was an integrated system, all one had to do in order to define it was to plot the geographic boundaries of the catchment area according to population, and to add measures of the appropriate subsystem.

Not only did this allow professionals to feel confident that their services were aiding "the community" by extending traditional services, but it also gave them an aura of social science respectability. Since the rhetoric of consensual systems dominated the literature of the social and behavioral sciences, its inclusion in community mental health seemed natural.

This system model also allowed professionally controlled services to address the issue of "community" by guiding administrators in the identification of appropriate subsystems to be connected with existing services. For example, community control could be discussed in terms of comprehensiveness of care, continuity of services, target populations, etc. [11]. It defined for those in control, the questions to be asked regarding the responsiveness of services to the "community." Their community would include the police, clergy, and schools—the subsystems of law, religion, education, in consensual language and issues of media coverage and bus service—the subsystems of communication and transportation. Any characteristic thus identified as part of the "system" could be translated into the domain of services for the franchise area. This consensual definition of community also limited the range of questions asked about services. It did not include emphasis on just who controlled what for whom within the community. It did not raise underlying questions of injustice in the given order of things. It did not necessitate a dynamic understanding of the history of social, cultural or economic networks. The idea that professional control of services might be limiting or inappropriate, or that system elements might be artificial creations developed by planners for their own ends, did not come into the consciousness of the general public until the late 1960s.

The tone of these early priestly writers was quietly subdued and restrained. There was no reason to use strong language and to spew forth polemics in order to convince readers that community was a system—what could be more obvious, more noncontroversial, more "scientific"? There was no strong talk of power and control of questioning "legitimate authorities," or of pushing for fundamental social change. The message was that experts could apply their specialized knowledge to define a geographic area and translate it into an administrative unit.

COMMUNITY AS CONSCIOUSNESS

Howe

A somewhat different orientation was developed out of the sociological consensual model by introduction of the concept of "community as collective consciousness," an idea presented in the landmark *Handbook of Community Psychiatry and Community Mental Health* published in 1964 and edited by Leopold Bellak [12].

The very first chapter of this text contained the work of a sociologist, Louisa Howe, who had both a Ph.D. in sociology and extensive psychiatric experience. Among other accomplishments, Dr. Howe had worked at the Menningers' Hospital, had trained in psychoanalysis in the Boston Psychoanalytic Institute and had numbered among her students Bertram Brown, later to become Head of NIMH. (Dr. Howe, into the 1990s, was to remain active in the practice of psychotherapy and in the Sociological Practice Association as a clinical sociologist.)

Dr. Howe's, "The Concept of the Community: Some Implications for the Development of Community Psychiatry," [13, pp. 16-64] presented the idea that community may be viewed as a "functional" community which was based on geography, (somewhat akin to the traditional consensual systems approach), or as a community based on functions of persons such as a community of doctors, or as "levels" of community including family, households, or cities, all dependent on ties of mutual interdependence.

Dr. Howe's own preference was for a definition of community [13, p. 19]:

> . . . as an analytic concept (in the logical sense), rather than to identify it with concretely existing aggregations of people. It can then be seen as a 'dimension' of human behavior, a 'component' of man's view of himself and his fellows.

In addition to this symbolic interactional view, Dr. Howe suggested that the concept would be most fruitfully applied through imagining community operating on a "symbolic" level consisting of a "sense of common destiny" [13, pp. 19-29]. This common destiny, Dr. Howe suggested, could be seen through the study of law and during times of heightened crisis and conflict [13, pp. 20-24].

This view might be seen as falling between a consensual ideal of shared values and a humanist class model based on common consciousness growing out of shared class positions, although Dr. Howe does not go so far as to invoke the concept of class. She did apply her "community" to the role of psychiatry, especially in terms of the work of psychiatrist as consultant to the community. In her discussion, she addressed questions such as: Whom the consultant should approach?, What questions should be asked?, and Which attitudes should be displayed? Most interesting in this discussion is the author's view of how to handle opposition to consultation. She stated that the psychiatrist may well have to act before everyone has decided to trust him and to accept his judgement.[1] Attacks, according to the author, may come from persons defending their community because they see dangers from the psychiatrist's action, or from certain persons "whose position is marginal to the main body of the community, and who are regarded by the community as 'deviant'" [13, p. 36]. Dr. Howe suggested that the psychiatrist accede with good grace to requests that are made of him by "accredited representatives of the community" [13, p. 36] and that, if

---

[1]Howe referred to therapists as males in these writings, as was the common practice of the time. She herself was one of the early women to attain a position in the inner-circle of influential mental health policy makers in the United States.

the psychiatrist foresees problems for the community, and informs "responsible people," then these "responsible community agents" will be grateful. As with other consensual works, the implication is that those defined as "legitimate authorities" in the community are therefore "responsible." Since, according to this author, the community is based on consensus as revealed through its common laws and sense of common destiny, marginals or deviants are those outside this common body—a clearly articulated priestly, consensual approach to defining deviance. The author goes on the state [13, p. 39]:

> It seems clear, furthermore, that mental or emotional 'disorder' signifies not only an 'illness' to be treated by a physician; it also expresses lack of order in the community.
> Rational order, under law, is upheld through the power of 'discourse' among free men, in Duncan's phrase; it depends upon the human capacities and social arrangements that make symbolic communication freely possible among members of a community.
> Nonrational order also exists and is based on hierarchical principles upheld by barriers of mystery that separate one group or class from another.

The psychiatrist must break down these barriers and open communication, supporting order. Here again the author has stated an assumption that value consensus forms the basis of community. The view that disorder, conflict, and failure to uphold consensus are intrinsically deviant falls quite clearly in the priestly, consensual tradition.

How did this author view "legitimate authorities?" In the summary of her article, the author stated that community members wherever they stood in the hierarchy of community, should be approached with deference and trust; that they should "be given a chance to look over the goods" [13, p. 41] and make up their own minds [13, p. 42].

> This sort of approach to those who represent the dominant sources of power in the community—particularly business and industrial leaders—can yield approval and sanction that help in overcoming skepticism at somewhat lower levels. . . . Perhaps the leading businessman in the community worries about his assistant manager, who is goofing off. The psychiatrist, meanwhile, is mainly concerned with patients. But if the businessman is helped to deal with his problem, chances are good that his perception will expand to include the psychiatrist's concerns as well.

Here the emphasis is placed on facilitating the functioning of the legitimate authorities, i.e. businessmen and industrial leaders, while meeting the therapeutic ends of the psychiatrist. If the psychiatrist can display social control skills in helping the businessman deal with an insubordinate assistant, then these same social control methods may win the psychiatric consultant entree into other territories controlled by community authorities. This was a practical and pragmatic approach to extending consultation practice.

Thus far, several models of community have been reviewed, including community as market, as catchment, as field and as collective consciousness. As has been suggested, the first two—community as market and as catchment area—complement each other by supporting professional dominance and translating easily into planning areas. The second two models, community as field and as collective consciousness, use the rhetoric of priestly, consensual social science. They rest on assumptions of consensually agreed upon norms and values, and they share a systems model of structure which implicitly legitimate persons in positions of power or authority. They adopt an evolutionary model of community change, and are written in mild, measured language.

One of the most important applications of the consensual model for the CMHC literature came from the innovative CMHC service of community consultation—an issue already presented in the writings of Howe and drawing on earlier, unpublished work by Erick Lindemann. Consultation, unlike the more traditional interventions of inpatient, outpatient, and emergency services, required the mental health workers to leave the medical/psychiatric environment and venture forth into the world outside of the clinic or hospital.

CONSULTATION: AGENTS OF COMMUNITY CHANGE?

In 1968 an insider's view at what was to be considered one of the most innovative aspects of the CMHC movement—community consultation—was published, *Mental Health Consultants, Agents of Community Change*, authored by Charles R. Griffith and Lester M. Libo [14]. The work recounted a program in the early 1960s which placed four mental health consultants in culturally diverse, rural and resource poor, geographically defined areas of New Mexico. The work is important not just because it was authored by two leading figures in the field of community mental health, but because it purported to document mental health consultants as agents of community change. This was a bold assertion.

The consultants came from a variety of professional backgrounds, but they worked under the direction of a psychiatrist. This reflected the norm of the period when psychiatrists directed CMHCs and were considered to be in charge of the mental illness treatment market.

The consultants included two Ph.D. clinical psychologists, a nurse mental health consultant with a masters degree and specialization in public health, and a masters level psychiatric social worker. These consultants were charged with the following: to cooperatively interact with existing mental health personnel and services; to offer guidance to community agencies interested in developing new services; to coordinate information; and to offer training to professional and lay persons. All services were overseen by the psychiatrist who traveled among districts and offered supervision.

This effort was importantly influenced by anthropological approaches to community which emphasized issues of culture. As Griffith and Libo wrote [14, p. 29]:

> In our conceptual framework, institutions, agencies, groups and even ideas within our society can be studied from a cultural perspective. There are agreed upon 'rules of the game' . . .

One concern was that the consultants might upset these cultural frameworks causing conflict to arise. Such organizational conflict was likened to a patient's conflict or crises which "lays bare conscious and unconscious motivations, goals, and philosophies, while consensus, although highly desirable, often leaves one satisfied but unenlightened" [14, p. 30].

In this sense the approach was within the ecological literature of the period, looking at the interwoven values which linked personal, family, and organizational structures within the community. As might be expected from professionals closely allied with the CMHC movement of the time, the phrase "agents of community change" referred chiefly to value structures influencing the existing mental illness treatment services rather than the larger sociocultural environment.

Community, although never specifically defined, was addressed by the project leaders in terms of the social and cultural characteristics of each district. The categories used in coding these characteristics for the methodology of the study were taken from the Human Relations Area Files. Among other variables, they included community power structure, economic behavior and organization, and sexual division of labor [14, p. 169]. Although these issues were mentioned in initial chapters of the book on the culture and history of the mental health districts, they did not seem to figure prominently in the conceptualization of the actual work of the consultants. In other words, the consultants, tasks did not seem to include modification of these infrastructural elements.

It is instructive to look at the data from the consultants' daily logs of their work to assess just how their role of community change agents was implemented. Although significant differences were seen between the activities of the nurse and social worker on one hand and the two clinical psychologists on the other, all four consultants spent most of their efforts on "expediting interagency communication, referrals, and community-wide coordination of services" [13, p. 130].

Conducting case consultation was the second most frequently cited activity. The authors note that although these activities were closely linked to the program's objectives, "such involvement with existing community agencies and their professional staffs tended to limit the consultants' visibility to the general public" [13, p. 130]. This is a particularly telling statement when one asks the question how these consultants could be termed agents of community change when the consultants spent most of their time with other professionals. A more apt term might have been agents on behalf of the development and networking of mental illness and mental retardation services.

The designers of the program codified the appropriate behavior for the consultants in their Project Coding Manual. Here "content of interaction" included such activities as getting acquainted with establishing rapport, providing mental health information services, and conducting mental health education and training programs with professional or lay groups. This last included a wide variety of civic organizations such as the American Legion, the Mental Health Association, the League of Women Voters and others. Missing from this coding list were the terms which later conflict theorists most probably would have considered as essential for addressing true community change, terms such as empowering disenfranchised persons and groups, reducing social inequality, and addressing alienation. Also missing were the groups which would have been considered as instrumental in achieving these goals, that is community-based activist groups dedicated to goals quite different from those of the mainstream civic organizations reached by the consultants.

The authors of the project did not ignore the impact of national politics on the work they documented. They acknowledged the change in the political climate relative to mental health between the late 1950s and the mid 1960s. The major lessons they drew from this change is one of growing interest in and funding for prevention, of increased public demand for services, and especially the rising interest in addressing unmet needs in services for the mentally retarded.

In their summary of the program's accomplishments, the authors linked these political changes closely to financing changes when they wrote [13, p. 175]:

> Perhaps the best measure of this improvement in public support is found in the budget of the Mental Health Division itself. From financing that was almost entirely federal, the Division has progressed to the point of enjoying the status accorded programs with earmarked budget items derived in large part from state funds.

The consultant's work is then credited with this "significant accomplishment in the history of New Mexico's public health mental health program" [13, p. 175]. This seems to be a clear statement that what are termed "agents of community change" during this early era of the CMHC movement were importantly agents of expanding and refining the political economy of professional mental illness services.

COMMUNITY ACTION AS CONSULTATION AND EDUCATION

Caplan

The literature on consultation had been growing since the 1950s, but came into its own during the late 1960s and early 1970s. As the Lounsbury et al., content analysis of articles in the *Community Mental Health Journal* revealed, in that one journal alone, articles dealing with consultation had gone from 7.5 percent of the total number of articles in 1965-1968, up to 11 percent in 1969-1972 [1, p. 272]. In addition, overall articles on consultation were the second most frequently mentioned topic in the journal, the first being general "think pieces."

Although there are several important figures, including Linderman and Vaughn [15] associated with consultation, along with many others [16, 17] the most esteemed and influential author on consultation was Gerald Caplan. Caplan took Erick Lindemann's old spot at the Harvard School of Public Health when Lindemann moved to become Chief of Psychiatry as the Massachusetts General Hospital. In the early 1950s Lindemann had established a program in Community Mental Health in the School of Public Health, the Program Caplan came to lead. Unlike Lindemann who published little while nonetheless exerting a tremendous influence on the discipline, Caplan published prodigiously and his writings had far-reaching influence. In the 1970s alone, Dr. Caplan's works were cited in *The Social Science Citation Index*, almost two hundred times. Perhaps his most influential work was his 1970 work, *The Theory and Practice of Mental Health Consultation* [18] to be discussed later.

In 1968, Dr. Caplan delivered an address to the Walter Reed Institute of Research in Washington detailing his "Conceptual Models in Community Mental Health." Published several years later in a collection of his works [19], Dr. Caplan wrote that this lecture represented "my model of models" [19, p. xvi]. Dr, Caplan claimed to be eclectic in his approach [19, p. xvi]:

> If we wish to operate in a sophisticated manner in a variety of situations, we therefore need to develop and refine a series of models that we utilize in a differentiated way to complement each other.

However, a closer sociological investigation reveals a rather sweeping consensual basis to his models, including his nutritional model, his developmental adjustment or crisis model, his community organization and development model, his socialization or effective role performance model. Consensualism is also evident in his models of practice encompassing a public health model practice model (including issues of epidemiology, catchment areas, planning and logistics, concepts of prevention), a medical practice of doctor/patient model, and ecological system model, and a model of shared professional domains.

Caplan's discussion of the community organization and development model starts with reference to the research of the Leightons on the development of a "community as a problem-solving organization," clearly implying the existence of community as an entity in and of itself. He writes [19, p. 248]:

> If the community has a well developed pattern of leaders and followers, good communications, and effective control system, and efficient ways of identifying problems and of mobilizing and deploying its resources to deal with them, as well as a value system which accepts the importance of satisfying the human needs of its members, it is likely that the prevalence of mental disorder will be lower than in a similar population and ecological setting which manifests a less developed communal problem solving structure.

The fit of this statement to the consensual ideal typical model presented earlier is somewhat startling. Caplan is suggesting that a healthy community, one which is an effective problem-solving organization, must have a well developed authority structure, an effective control system, and a dominant value system which identifies needs of its members. In the language of the consensual model these notions would translate to a community having a legitimate authority system, sanctions and socialization carried out by those authorities, and a foundation built on value consensus. No mention is made by Caplan of competing leaders, competing value systems, and competing control systems.

Caplan goes on to suggest that this community model provides [19, p. 248]:

> ... a guide for all types of prevention of mental disorder through nonspecific community development, which focuses on the recruitment and training of leaders, improving communication, and helping to work out effective ways of organizing the people so that they learn how to identify salient problems and to mobilize internal and external resources in grappling with them.

Here again the assumption is that by recruiting and training leaders the community as an entity will be made healthier. There is no analysis of historically based competing leaders, clashes of interests, or oppositional classes. Nor is there mention as to whether "mobilizing resources" may mean mobilizing resources of one particular group over and against another. If such questions were addressed within a conflict model, it might be seen that mobilizing resources can further heighten class antagonisms and lead to breakdown in "legitimate authority," and communication.

Caplan next presents a model of socialization or effective role performance. Here he writes [19, p. 249]:

> ... mental disorder is seen as a condition of deviant functioning in an individual who does not conform to social expectations or appropriate behavior in his roles as a member of his family, work, social, cultural and religious groups. This deviance is often caused by his inability for a variety of reasons to occupy those roles, and by the ineffectiveness of the usual network of expectations and sanction in modeling his behavior, as well as by the concurrence of this social milieu in supporting his deviant behavior.

This could well have been written by Talcott Parsons. Caplan discusses "the role" as if it were consensually agreed upon, and supported its integration into the social system. As with Parsons, Caplan sees the family, work, religious groups, all supporting the normative pattern. No mention is made of the possibility of competing social expectations or of their limiting aspects. The question of whether family, work, religious conviction, etc., might themselves serve a larger socio-economic or political process is not raised.

Caplan says this model [19, p. 249]:

> . . . provides a guide to re-educational or re-socializing ways of bringing the deviant back into line with a socially productive and self-satisfying set of roles in the community. Instead of the disordered person being defined as sick and needing medical treatment in a hospital or clinic administered by a physician, he is seen as a student, apprentice, or trainee, who must be involved in an educational or training program administered and staffed by educators and vocational or industrial training specialists. Issues such as communication, motivation and control, by reward and punishment, material and methods of learning, and individual or group reinforcement become salient, as do ways of organizing training establishments which optimize the fit between current and future individual capacity, and social and occupation demands.

Here the author's faith in the existence of a consensually agreed upon "socially productive and self-satisfying set of rules in the community" is reiterated. The individual failing to conform to these is seen as a legitimate target for resocialization, group pressure, and education. No question is asked as to the motivation of non-conforming behavior. No mention is made of who is defining "current and future individual capacity," or whether "social and occupational demands" might not serve one group rather than another with equal claim.

Armed with these conceptual tools, consultants serving CMHC's took to the "community" during this era to spread the good word about preventive mental health. There was usually little question as to the proper target for such messages. As Caplan himself wrote in 1970 in *The Theory and Practice of Mental Health Consultation*, "In this book the term 'consultation' is used in a quite restrictive sense to denote a process of interaction between two professional persons . . ." [18, p. 19]. And later [18, pp. 20-21]:

> The consultees are drawn from the ranks of those care giving professionals, who, as mentioned previously, play a major role in preventing or testing mental disorders but who customarily have no specialized training in psychiatry and its allied disciplines. They include family doctors, pediatricians, and other medical specialists

such as obstetricians, internists, and surgeons, hospital and public health nurses, teachers, clergymen, lawyers, welfare workers, probation officers, and policemen.

Conspicuous by their absence are "non-legitimate authorities" including persons engaged in social change efforts or ordinary citizens, rather than those employed to maintain the ruling or dominant authority line.

A clear view of the author's model of community can be gleaned from his suggestions for explorations of the community to establish goals of consultation. Two aspects of the goals of the consultation are important; namely, salience, i.e., rank-ordering goals in regard to their importance in the current feelings of need in the community (here note is given to increasing communication skills for those hidden away but possibly in greatest need, so that those at the mental health agency can judge the consequences to the mental health picture of the community if the need is not met); and judging the importance of the goal in the overall mission of the agency. Here the author is aware of the historical changes which directly influence what is defined as important by those in charge [18, p. 41].

> It must be recognized that a judgement on the salience of a goal is relatively arbitrary, involving, as it does, a complicated tangle of factors. It is particularly susceptible to influence by the spirit and value system of the times and by fashions in professional style. These will, in turn, reflect both long term and short term historical trends. For instance, despite all the available evidence that mental disorder was most pressing among the poor and was so widespread as to over burden all efforts at direct professional action, it was not till the 1960s that it became fashionable within the framework of the antipoverty campaign to focus specialized mental health attention on metropolitan slums, and to do so with self-help and supports of prevention and remedial action by the poor themselves.

Several important points are contained within this paragraph. Although the author acknowledges the multifaceted nature of determining the salience of goals for the agency and the community, he seems to suggest that there is indeed a "value system" in place reflecting both short and long-term historical trends. Rather than positing several competing value systems or the interrelationship between authorities and these values, the implication seems to be that the value system has been developed as the outcome of the historical trends. The example mentioned, of combining mental health work with anti- poverty programs, is illustrative, because here the assumption is that for some reason in the 1960s it became fashionable to combine them. The fact that mental health programs were funded by the State during this period is not specifically linked to the possibility of social control or maintaining the dominant value system along with the aid of psychiatrists.

Rather than developing an alternative analysis, the author goes on to comment on the feasibility of goals set. He suggests that the effectiveness of intervention depends somewhat on the susceptibility to change manifested by the particular person or group. "Systems are more susceptible to change and more open to outside influence during periods of disequilibrium" [18, p. 42]. Here the concept is clearly taken from system models of society; a community in disequilibrium is more susceptible to consultation for change. The idea that disequilibrium, conflict, and change are endemic to the given system, are in fact is basic social process, is not considered. The example given by Caplan of an experience of disequilibrium is the rioting occurring in the late 1960s. The question addressed is the relationship of the mental health workers to the police during such a period. Caplan notes that mental health workers might experience dissonance with the values and actions of police during periods of unrest and, therefore, be unhappy about allying themselves with them. But his analysis of the situation is made clearer when he suggests that current events, such as the change of a mayor or a new police commissioner, might change the situation significantly and clear up the initial dissonance. Obviously, the author is not assuming that there exists any perpetual conflict between dominant and non-dominant groups in society. The question is more one of assessing the situation in a time of passing disequilibrium. As Caplan writes [18, p. 42]:

> Mental health planners and organizers must therefore be continually alert to the probable ripple effects of changes that satisfy the felt need of certain people and fit in with their own agency mission and professional concepts. What will be the inevitable opposition? Whose comfort will be upset? Whose rights will be threatened? Can this damage be overcome or minimized? Will the cost of the side effects be worth the central achievement?

From these questions, it certainly seems that Caplan is aware of the politics of change. He clearly know that changes among one group might well call forth opposition elsewhere and that consultants must see both the short and long-term political repercussions of their action on the community and their agency. Yet, what continues to be missing is any statement linking interests to ongoing historical processes, linking State authorities and agents of control to such processes, and plotting the position of the professional psychiatrists in all of this. The systems model simply obscures endemic conflict since the implication is of mutually reciprocal exchanges among subsystems which brings the system back to stability. Authorities, it is assumed, are consensually agreed upon in order to maintain stability of values and power.

The most vivid statement of Caplan's view on these issues comes in the last chapter of the book, a chapter entitled, "Mental Health Consultation and Community Action." In these last twenty-eight pages of the book, Caplan changes both content and tone. It is interesting to note that the author, in the beginning of the work, states he had been writing the book over several decades, and this last part had only just been written in the last few years. The passion of the times is quite obvious in the tone of this last part. From lengthy discussions of consultation, using verbatim reports of interviews, Caplan switches the focus of his thoughts to the macro-political context of consultation. He recounts the impact of the consumer revolt, including groups as diverse as "students, patients, the poverty stricken, the socially disadvantaged, Negroes, and other minority groups" [18, p. 353]. They are, he writes, expressing their dissatisfaction with the planning and implementation of community programs. This revolt, as he perceives it, is often turbulent because of [18, p. 354],

> . . . the buildup of past frustrations and angry disappointments, and because of the absence of a common semantic framework and a traditionally developed structure within which the two sides can communicate freely and negotiate peaceably.

Here, Caplan stresses the need to communicate, to share semantic frameworks, which he sees as the key to resolving these disputes.

This interpretation is reinforced when Caplan writes that consumers are rebelling precisely because they have not secured their rights, as they see them, through the orderly process designed and administered by the organizers of the community institutions and services. "Moreover, large segments of public opinion accept the notion that disadvantaged groups perceive different needs for themselves than do the professionals and experts and that the former's perception is apt to be more authentic" [18, p. 354]. Does this mean that Caplan acknowledges ongoing and irreconcilable differences between the needs of these groups and the "legitimate authorities?" Only in the sense that liberal reformers do so, without having to abandon their consensual model [18, p. 354].

> The right of the disadvantaged to maximum feasible satisfaction of basic needs is now beginning to be accepted as a fundamental axiom of our national life. From this, it follows that until an orderly process can be worked out for meaningful participation of consumers in the organization of services that cater to them, we must expect a transitional period of disorderly confrontation between consumers and providers of services.

But what is the method for satisfying the basic human needs of all citizens and what is this endpoint to which the current transitional phase is leading? It is highly doubtful that Caplan is writing about, for example, a transition to a socialist form of government or about any fundamental transformation in the socio-political structure. Rather he is stating his belief that, when equilibrium is restored, when services are open to all on an equitable basis and lines of communication are opened within the present system, then the system will again function smoothly.

Until such a time, mental health consultants will have to question for whom they are working and toward what end. As Caplan has pointed out, consultants are by far most frequently working for establishment agents [18, p. 355].

> Usually, however, there is no legitimated role for mental health workers as advocates for the consumer population, nor have they any status acceptable to both sides as mediators or arbitrators in trying to resolve the conflict between an institution and its clients.

The reason that consultants are habitually seen as agents of the establishment, and not acceptable as mediators, is, to Caplan, an issue of carving out roles, explaining and demonstrating neutrality, simply acting as facilitators of consensus rather than purveyors of the dominant culture [18, p. 355].

> It may take ten to fifteen years to work out an orderly procedure to involve recipient populations in the planning and management of service program that cater to them, and to provide acceptable mechanisms with which to deal smoothly with the discrepancies that inevitably occur. I believe that eventually such procedures and mechanisms will be developed, just as they have been in the somewhat analogous field of labor-management conflicts.

Again the issue is one of providing mechanisms for voicing grievances and holding hearings—facilitating communication. The issue of overturning the system itself, of facilitating heightened conflict simply to fuel the inevitable change process, to put the consumer in charge completely in a totally new power structure, is not addressed.

The judgement of the consultant must be used to decide whether to work as an ally of his/her institution, as an ally of the consumer for both the institution and the consumer, and/or as a mediator [18, p. 358]:

> . . . owing primary allegiance to neither side but trusted by both to safeguard their interests to the maximum possible degree and to assist each to clarify the priorities of its demands and then to negotiate an agreement by mutual trade-offs.

This statement again reflects the belief of the author that, after all, these consumer demands are negotiable within the given system. If one were putting forth a conflict theory analysis, these demands would be seen as reflecting emergent class consciousness and, as such, would be incompatable with the needs and desires of the dominant group.

What would be the alternative conflict model of mental health consultations? The collaborators defined through a conflict model would not be legitimate authorities as defined by the professionals, nor would they be the professionals themselves, unless they were specifically allied with the non-dominant group. They would be leaders of the opposition or members of minorities of working class movements historically opposed to the establishment which hires and pays most, if not all, of what Caplan considers potential mental health consultants. Expertise on interactional processes, human motivations, planning techniques would be shared by mental health consultants with those seeking to change, fundamentally, the structure of the social system. The model informing such sharing of information would not be a consensual systems model which is a model based on the assumed legitimacy of policy, teachers, clergy, etc. A conflict model would be based on improving the unity of emergent class consciousness. A conflict analyst would replace the consensual emphasis on communication with an alternative emphasis on empowerment of oppositional elements. A conflict analyst would also replace the consensual emphasis on equilibrium with an alternative emphasis on heightened discord and preparing the way for the emergence of a new liberated order. The path to establishing this new structure was not completely defined in the conflict literature, but the struggle to define it was at the heart of the conflict approach. Authors such as Gorz [20] had a decade earlier begun explorations along this path by differentiating reforms which created heightened structural tensions from those which did not. Following this path would lead consultants to explore ways in which their skills could support appropriate points of significant structural change. Consultation would not automatically be supportive of the given authority structure, but it would be guided by an explicit analysis of power and control, of class and class interests in a given historical setting. Such analysis would directly involve uniting the skills of conflict sociologists with those of psychiatric experts.

Does any of this come into play in Caplan's actual practice? Are there points at which a conflict model emerges in his writing? Answers are supplied by the following analysis of the last chapter of his work, *The Theory and Practice of Mental Health Consultation*, the case study of a mental health consultant who was present during confrontations between an organized group of blacks involved with a school and the school administration.

CONFLICT OR CONSENSUS? CAPLAN'S CASE

We are told that the case concerns a mental health center in a city of 300,000. A psychiatric consultant from a community mental health center is working with a school principal who heads a school in the middle of a poor, black neighborhood. The shy, middle-aged white principal is consulting with the psychiatrist when an angry group of black parents forces its way into his office. The CMHC consultant offers his help in regard to a meeting between the parents and the principal which is set to be held in several weeks. During the meeting, at which the consultant sits quietly near the principal, the principal tires to assure the audience that he has taken the correct steps in relaying their demands to the administrative authorities. The parents react angrily, saying they have waited too long already. Then, as the author states [18, p. 361]:

> At this stage, a new element was added to the meeting. Two men in the audience who were not parents but black community militants, became active in the discussion. They spoke in a hostile and insulting way to the principal and school staff, calling the latter a 'pack of white-assed bitches' and stirring up the rest of the audience to join in their attacks, which became increasingly more ugly. The principal and a couple of teachers attempted to defend

themselves and engage in rational discussion, but they were shouted down and the meeting broke up in disorder.

The consultant spent two hours with the principal and staff, "helping them regain their poise and understand what happened" [18, p. 361]. He pointed out that the local issues involved the legitimacy of some of the demands and explained how the meeting was being overpowered by the tensions in the black community, "It seemed as though Black Power activists were exploiting the situation as an opportunity to bring a basic black-white conflict into the open" [18, p. 361]. The consultant's suggestion was to bring higher authorities into the picture and to depend on the mental health center as a resource. Back at the mental health center, the consultant discussed the next development which was a message conveyed through the principal that the district superintendent did not want to get involved. This was followed by a quiet period of several months interrupted only by sporadic incidents at the school. At the end of the school year, a center staff person who held a meeting with the district superintendent found him talking only about individual problems of emotionally disturbed or educationally backward children.

The next school year brought an outbreak of conflict when a new principal at the school refused to meet with a group of parents. That group marched into the school yard where they were confronted by the police. Meanwhile, a Freedom School was set up in a community recreational building by a parent's committee.

At this point, a five-member committee of black and white professionals from the ghetto called on the center director, asking him to help resolve the situation before it got totally out of hand. They felt that the main problem revolved around the school authorities' refusal to meet with the parents and to discuss their legitimate demands; and they placed particular blame on the new school principal, who was making matters worse by his high-handed authoritarian approach to the parents [18, p. 363].

The outcome of this meeting was that the center set up a meeting with the school officials including the deputy superintendent. That official voiced the opinion that the situation was not the business of the psychiatric consultant since his expertise was with troubled children [18, p. 365].

> The director replied that his center was concerned with all community issues that might affect the sense of well-being of children and their families and that might be conductive to mental

health or mental disorder. He felt that racial tensions and lack of consonance between parents and educators must inevitably affect the feeling of security of many families and might have a deleterious effect on the emotional stability of school children. Moreover, problems of communication between individuals and groups were a topic of special interest to mental health specialists and one in which they had developed some expert knowledge.

He also told the superintendents that his visitors had predicted a more dangerous community upheaval if the local problem between the ghetto school and the parent's group was not quickly resolved. He said that the center staff, like all citizens, had a fundamental interest in preserving public order and preventing damage to property and lives, such as had recently occurred in their cities as a consequence of similar racial conflict in the schools.

At this, the superintendent warmly welcomed the help of the consultants, reporting that the parents had been making a "series of outrageous demands," most of which couldn't be dealt with in practical terms. . . . For example, they wanted complete community control over the school with power to hire and fire its personnel. They demanded a black principal. They wanted several of their number to be put on the school payroll as 'guardians of discipline' in the school" [18, p. 365]. The principal wanted to talk with the parents and engage them in "rational discussion." However, the tale of former meetings, including insults and rage from the black community, had stiffled their feeling that rationality was possible. The school officials felt that school disruptions and the Freedom School were the work of "outside agitators." Criminal charges were discussed. The school officials and the mental health center decided on a plan to negotiate with a community leader, if one could be found, "whose prestige would place him above the frey."

After this, a series of meetings with the mayor and the choosing of a group to represent the parents, a group which had to be distinguished enough to be acceptable by the school officials, occupied the consultant's time. The reluctance of the mayor to get involved and the haggling over the membership of the negotiating group stymied the intentions of the center to speed high level negotiations. The mayor finally appointed his own group to study the situation over a protracted period of time. This angered the center's director who set up his own meeting between school officials and black representatives. The initially amicable atmosphere of this meeting turned into open hostility when the parent's committee chairman read a written statement of demand from the group. The center's leader appealed for order. "The center director's appeal was successful, and the final few minutes of the discussion reverted to friendly rationality" [18, p. 370]. This was followed by a series of three more meetings, all erupting into hostility [18, p. 371].

> It became clear that part of the difficulty in communication was caused by the parents' oversimplified view of the school system. The center director drew this point to the attention of both sides and emphasized the necessity, in order to ensure meaningful communication, of their learning the cognitive framework that each was using.

The negotiations seemed to break down completely. The center director was now perceived by the black leaders to "be an agent of the school department" and no further meetings were scheduled.

The case description ends rather abruptly with the final page of Caplan's fourteen page report. He concluded suddenly, "the ice was broken," and through a series of secret meetings between the parents and the school officials held at the center, a mutually satisfactory agreement was reached. "The Freedom School was disbanded, and all the children were brought back to the ghetto school" [18, p. 372].

The center staff was happy since they felt they had cooled down an inflammatory situation, allowing both sides to overcome obstacles to communication and to negotiate a settlement [18, p. 373].

> As this negotiation got under way, the participants became able to focus effectively on their real problems and to prevent outsiders from exploiting them for the satisfaction of their own political needs."

The report ends with a statement that the whole series of encounters had strengthened the relationship of the center with the school, although the black community now identified the CMHC as "part of the services of the school department and not as an acceptable advocate for their side" [18, p. 372]. The last sentence reads, "It was difficult to determine how the black community had perceived the center before its intervention in this conflict, and how this image had been affected, if at all, by this operation" [18, p. 372].

From a prophetic, conflict perspective this case is indeed telling. It began with a typical meting between social control agents, a psychiatrist and a school principal, who were confronted by demands from a group of black parents. Not surprisingly, the psychiatrist decided to offer his help by supporting the principal's effort to communicate. What might have been defined as attempts at reallocating power, was defined instead as nonrational and inappropriate hostility, the results of misunderstandings which hindered rational communication. From the point of view of the school officials, "extreme demands," such as control of the school and the hiring of community members as control agents, were seen as the work of outside militants. This clearly mirrors the opposing world views of the dominant versus the nondominant group. The parents' view of the school is seen as "oversimplified," a statement which reflects the mystification of bureaucracy which in itself is a control tactic. The involvement of higher and higher authorities was seen as a way to resolve the conflict since involvement was supposed to facilitate the communication flow and to re-equilibrate the dysfunctional cycle of anger and frustration.

The mental health consultant continued to perceived this facilitation of communication as the key to resolving the situation. As the center director himself pointed out to the school officials, mental health consultants could facilitate communication, thereby averting riots which were detrimental to the mental health of the children in the community. The transformation of the psychiatrist consultant role from being an expert on pathology in children to becoming an expert in communications for community groups was accepted because the consensual systems model legitimated the standing of the school authorities. If communication was the key, no one in authority would lose power or control; no basic changes would be made. Everyone would eventually see the "truth," and the truth would prevail over "hotheads."

The attempt to involve the State directly in the person of the mayor was ineffective, since his adopted role as mediator between warring class factions prevented action. Perched precariously between two adversarial groups, his inaction was based on the correct perception of the real incompatibility of the power demands of the blacks and the existing system represented by the school. Interestingly enough, the psychiatrists were the ones with enough flexibility to cool out the parents' group and restore the control of the existing system.

Ironically, the consultants viewed communication difficulties as being at the heart of the failure to negotiate. This conclusion contradicted their own realization of the actual demands of the black parents, demands clearly enough understood in their implication to be labelled irrational or the result of ignorance of the system.

Had the CMHC psychiatrists been operating from a conflict model, they might have first allied themselves with the black militants and offered support and skills from the other side of the table. They then would have had to confront inconsistencies in their own systems of value and authority. The outcome of this probably would have been disengagement of the center from activities it formerly supported such as work with police, some clergy, medical facilities, etc. In other words, to cross the line to the opposition would have meant attack from mainstream sources of support. Nonetheless, this course of action might have heightened tensions and precipitated meaningful change in the form demanded by the blacks including increased control of the school.

This example clarifies the implicit sociological model which informed consultation by reflecting choices based on the model of community, in this case a thoroughly priestly, consensual one. The model assumed that integration of subsystems was to be achieved through better communication, that traditional legitimate authorities were the ones to remain in control and that the State was to mediate disputes to return the system to equilibrium.

Caplan's text ended with a series of questions to himself and to his readers. How can the consultant help the underprivileged to achieve their goals?, to understand the system and to change it?, to exercise appropriate control over the hostile feelings of oppositional groups?, etc. Although these questions remained unanswered for Caplan, he found himself having to address the content of mass-based social movements [18, p. 381].

> What role should community mental health workers play in regard to this approach? Must we inevitably be on the side of conflict resolution by facilitating rational communication between parties to local disputes, or is there also a role for us in aiding the revolutionary forces that seek the destruction of systems in order to produce a fundamental improvement in the lot of the underprivileged populations? When I describe the behavior of the deputations . . . as 'irrational', is this not an expression of my biased identification with the system that prescribed the rules and seeks to force the recipients of care to communicate in a mode that inevitably gives the care giver officials the ship hand? In behaving violently and intemperately and in expressing the hostile feelings of their constituents, are the leaders not acting most sensibly, and should we be trying to cool them off? If we succeed, are we not helping to perpetuate the bad system, apart from a few minor changes?

Neither Caplan nor the other consensual theorists find answers to these troubling questions in their models. At best, they strove for corrections in what they perceived as the dysfunctions in the system. Perhaps the most surprising aspect of Caplan's analysis was not that answers to these questions were put off for the future, but that the questions were raised at all.

In the next chapter, rather different answers are presented when the conflict model emerges in the professional literature. It should be mentioned at this point that answers from a conflict perspective were also emerging in cross national psychiatry. Most academic psychiatrists and even academic anthropologists with whom they worked, such as Leighton [21] had little interest in studying explicitly political economic issues. These authors focused attention almost totally on the milder, priestly issues of community function. Questions as to the role of mental health workers in supporting or opposing given power structures were rarely questioned. The works of Frantz Fanon, published in the late 1960s, provided an analysis of psychiatry's role in colonial domination. These works seemed to have been a cry in the wilderness. Even by the end of the decade, such mainstream authors as Caplan had not moved to see the connection with what was being called internal colonialism and the black experience.

This reflects one of the most important lessons of this analysis—that priestly writers remained priests throughout the movement and that prophets remained prophets. At best, the dialogue called for by sociologists of knowledge such as Friedrichs [22] was achieved only in the sense that questions asked by the other side were appearing in priestly writings, albeit, with no answers.

REFERENCES

1. J. W. Lounsbury, K. G. Roeseim, L. Pokorny, A. Sills, G. J. Meissen, An Analysis of Topic Areas Trends in the *"Community Mental Health Journal"* from 1965 through 1977, *Community Mental Health Journal, 15*:9, pp. 267-276, 1979.

2. A Reference to Bernard L. Bloom, *Community Mental Health: A Historical and Critical Analysis*, General Learning Corp., Morristown, New Jersey, 1973.

3. F. J. Braceland, *Testimony in Support of Appropriations for the National Institute of Mental Health*, Subcommittee on Appropriations, U.S. Senate, Congressional Record, June 15, 1961.

4. United States Senate Subcommittee on Health, Mental Illness and Retardation, *Hearings before the Subcommittee on Health of the Committee on*

Labor and Public Welfare, U.S. Senate, 88th Congress, 1st Session, in S. 755 and 756, March 5, 6, 7, U.S. Govt. Printing Office, Washington, D.C., 1963.

5. B. Bloom, *Community Mental Health: A General Introduction*, Brooks/Cole, Monterey, California, 1977.

6. Joint Information Service, *The Community Mental Health Center: An Interim Appraisal*, Joint Information Service, Washington, D.C., 1969.

7. F. Perlmutter and H. Silverman, CMHC: A Structural Anachronism, *Social Work, 17*:2, pp. 78-84, 1972.

8. C. C. Huffine and T. J. Craig, Catchmenting and Community, *Archives of General Psychiatry, 28*, pp. 483-488, April, 1974.

9. D. C. Klein, The Community and Mental Health: An Attempt at a Conceptual Framework, *Community Mental Health Journal, 1*, pp. 301-308, 1965.

10. D. C. Klein, *Community Dynamics and Mental Health*, John Wiley & Sons, New York, 1968.

11. M. B. Smith and N. Hobbs, The Community and the Community Mental Health Center, *American Psychologist, 21*, pp. 299-309, 1966.

12. L. Bellak (ed.), *Handbook of Community Psychiatry and Community Mental Health*, Grune and Stratton, New York, 1964.

13. L. Howe, The Concept of Community, in *Handbook of Community Psychiatry and Community Mental Health*, L. Bellak, (ed.), Grune and Stratton, New York, pp. 16-64, 1964.

14. C. Griffith and L. M. Libo, *Mental Health Consultants: Agents of Community Change*, Jossey-Bass Company, San Francisco, 1968.

15. J. R. Ewalt and P. L. Ewalt, History of the Community Psychiatry Movement, *American Journal of Psychiatry, 126*, pp. 43-52, 1969.

16. American Psychological Association, Task Force on Community Issues, *Community Psychology and Preventive Mental Health*, Behavioral Press, New York, 1971.

17. M. M. Laurence, *The Mental Health Team in the Schools*, Behavioral Press, New York, 1971.

18. G. Caplan, *The Theory and Practice of Mental Health Consultation*, Basic Books, New York, 1970.

19. G. Caplan, Conceptual Models in Community Mental Health, Chapter 10 in *Support Systems and Community Mental Health*, Behavioral Publications, New York, 1974.

20. A. Gotz, *Socialism and Revolution*, Anchor Books, New York, 1973.

21. A. Leighton, *My Name Is Legion*, Basic Books, New York, 1959.

22. R. W. Friedrichs, *A Sociology of Sociology*, Free Press, New York, 1970.

CHAPTER 6

Theory during Phase Two when Conflict Emerges, the Mid 1960s to the Early 1970s

By the second half of the decade, neither academics not politicians could avoid acknowledging the social and political upheavals which surrounded them. The CMHC movement had been defined and directed by a special group of public health psychiatrists who had been allied with key administrators and with leaders in cooperating professions. Its promise of community mental health, and its link to funded reform movements such as vocational rehabilitation, children's services, poverty programs, housing and urban renewal made it a natural target for black power groups and other social change activists.

By 1967, these influences were being reflected in the more socially conscious mental health publications. For example, the *American Journal of Orthopsychiatry*, covered such topics in its pages as social responsibility in treating blue-collar workers, socio-psychiatry for the disadvantaged, commitment to peace work, and the war on poverty. The lead editorial for the index issue of that year was written by the co-chairs of the annual program committee and was entitled, "Mental Health is a Social Problem" [1]. In the next few years, radical caucuses of the American Psychiatric Association disrupted annual meetings with pie throwing and other demonstrations, and carried their demands from the streets into the inner circle of psychiatry.

As Duhn and Leopold wrote in 1969 [2], within those few years after the initial CMHC funding it became evident that events had outstripped even the original legislation. The riots, the crisis of the cities, and other social events, indicated the need for psychiatry to sensitized to political change. In the same year, H. Stuart Hughes delivered the Benjamin Rush lecture on the history of psychiatry before the 125th anniversary meeting of the American Psychiatric Association [3]. In this speech Hughes discussed the sense of dismay many felt: "We have become bewildered and resentful; we feel trapped and desperate" [3, p. 21]. Mentioning Vietnam, political assassinations, squalor and fear in ghettos, disappointment and disillusionment over Czechoslovakia, the author traced the silent generation of the 1950s as it gave way to the alienated generation of the 1960s. Warning his audience about the dangers of giving way to a new McCarthy era, of seeing all society as sick, Hughes reminded them that psychiatry had grown out of the liberal tradition and must stay there [3, p. 21].

Responding also to these conditions and events were academics in the conflict tradition, radical scholars who dismissed liberalism as bandaid reform. These conflict scholars also acknowledged the impact of changing political conditions on their scholarly work. As Colfax and Roach, editors of a volume entitled *Radical Sociology*, wrote [4, p. 19]:

> In four years, government repression of resistance to its genocidal policies has gone from the use of tear gas against Pentagon demonstrators to the shooting of college students. In the months since we first began to draw this volume together, politically motivated federal indictments have become commonplace, draft and Dow chemical file burners have been given long sentences for the destruction of property, the two mother-country revolutionary movements—Weatherman and Black Panther Party—have been destroyed and torn by factional fights, respectively, students in Kent State and Jackson have been murdered, thousands have died in Southeast Asia, and the Vietnam War is now the Indo-China War.

Clearly social control, both through overt force and through "ideological guidance," had spread from urban black movements to diverse and dispersed protest movements across the nation. Around the world, as well, political economic upheavals mounted. Protests about colonial wars in Algeria and elsewhere, as well as the war in Vietnam helped catalyze student rebellions in France, for example. The worldwide impact sent waves of reaction to the heart of the core capitalist nations.

In the United States, these events tended to polarize academics as well as the general public. Academics in the CMHC movement already

found themselves negotiating the shifting sands between individualistic models of psychopathology which supported capitalist ideologies
[5] and collectivistic models of social pathology which called forth new
models of care [6]. As the Health Policy Action Committee, an activist
health group in New York, wrote in 1969 [7, p. 2]:

> Does community mental health mean bringing traditional ser-
> vices to the community—or working on all fronts for a 'healthy'
> community? The Professionals who have ridden the Federal-
> funding wave into the streets are sharply divided. One camp see
> themselves, like Albert Schweitzer, establishing psychotherapeutic
> outposts in the jungle. Others see themselves as the vanguard in a
> trailblazing sweep through our urban wastelands—attacking poor
> housing, unemployment and all the other symptoms of a failing
> society. It is hard to say which approach is the most arrogantly
> ambitious, for it is not easier to cure individuals who live in a sick
> society than it is to 'treat' a society whose members have lost hope.

The Albert Schweitzers, those I have called traditionalists holding
to market, catchment area and consensual models, saw their mission
as spreading their services to needy patients in the community. The
trailblazers, more often than not liberal reformers voicing mixtures of
consensual and conflict models, saw their task as correcting the community, either through reforms or revolution. The possibilities for
change seemed unlimited, and the result was a new immediacy about
change which added vigor to the tone of the CMHC literature. The
literature took on the character of a cause, heartfelt and devoid of the
rather dry, rationalistic language of the early years. Now words of
passion conveyed issues of power and struggle. By the end of the
decade, the movement had won the title of a "boundaryless system"
from sociologists Dinitz and Beran [8]. The search for change had taken
psychiatrists to the edge of their traditional roles, and had fostered a
view that psychopathology had to be defined and treated within the
political economic context. As these authors wrote [8, p. 107]:

> Thus, community mental health, a boundaryless system, seems
> to have set for itself a boundaryless goal: the improvement of the
> quality of life of the whole man, and everyman, in his total environ-
> ment. In this role, community mental health appears to stand as
> a hallmark of the contemporary heightened awareness of the
> unbounded nature of our environment ills. Concern about clinical
> pathologies shares the limelight with concern about social and
> physical problems. Contaminants of all types are coming under
> heavy attack from many sectors; ameliorative efforts are being

directed against everything from emotional disorders, to racial tensions, to air and water pollution.

Traditional roles and models were clearly being stretched and molded to new demands [9].

This transformation brings to mind what Freidrichs [10] described as the difference between "priestly" and "prophetic" sociology. The rationalistic, supposedly value free, orientation of administrators and bureaucrats gave way to calls for action by angry young change agents. Rather than fitting the more traditional mold of a social movement, starting with ideological fervor and progressing into bureaucratic institutionalization, this movement seemed to catch fire in its middle years, the late 1960s, when American society itself be ablaze. Both sides, conservative traditionalists and radical reformers, developed strong models and vigorous rhetoric.

What was the meaning of "community" for community mental health authors now? Were they to wait and work for the emergence of class consciousness, for the community to march up to the center and take control as suggested by conflict theorists? Were they to take an enlightened liberal view toward organizing the community with the help of experts, such as Caplan, a consensual stance? Or were they to concentrate on developing and applying social indicators to community process in the hope of scientifically defining patients and community representatives, an administrative-planning stance?

CONFLICT EMERGES IN THE THEORY

By 1968 and 1969 the answers and the models were emerging in recognizable fashion. For conflict theorists, such as those reviewed in the following pages, the struggle over power and control united academics with street fighters. The battle over Lincoln Hospital and other such facilities had brought to the fore coalitions of academics and street gangs, such as the Young Lords, to discuss issues of "community control." No longer was this a polite discussion among academics about the supply of traditional services, but rather it was nitty-gritty detailing of who was to control what for whom [11].

Issues of Praxis and Control: Jonas

One of the best examples of this discussion was presented by Steven Jonas in an article for the *American Journal of Public Health* entitled, "A Theoretical Approach to the Question of 'Community Control' of

Health Facilities" published in 1971 [12]. In this work the issue most clearly addressed was change and control. The question of who constituted the community, who set standards and maintained the order, were not raised. Rather, the heart of the analysis was short-term and long-term strategies for control of the health care system in the United States.

Jonas almost immediately asked, "Where Does Control of Health Services Lie?" [12, p. 917]. In his answer he suggested that the building blocks of health service institutions were its capital structures, its expense budget, and the quantity and quality of its staff. The health care system, on the other hand, was based on its own organization, its financing, and its patterns of practice. Control of the building blocks of the institutions resided with the State, the President, the Congress, state government, and local officials. These, in turn, responded to industrial leaders, bankers, heads of major universities and foundations. Those elites determined finances, training, priorities, and all other vital issues concerning health care. Jonas argued that confrontations over administrative issues of hiring and firing were not issues of community control, but rather issues of community administrations, and therefore could not produce more than minor changes.

He also examined "the struggle for community control" as it related to the broader struggles for major social changes then under way in the United States [12, p. 919].

> Let it be assumed for the moment that to remove from American society such negative elements as involvement in the unpopular war in Vietnam, racism, the alienation of people from one another and from their work, environmental pollution, unemployment, and production for purposes other than use, that major social change will be necessary. Let it be assumed further that to achieve this major social change, the control over the ordering of national priorities and the distribution of national resources will have to be removed from the hands of those who have it now and put into other hands. Let it be assumed finally that to accomplish this transfer of power will require struggle. If those assumptions are correct, it would appear that the struggle for community control is diversionary and actually retrogressive.

The elements of conflict analysis were clearly presented. The focus was on an elite group controlling priorities (an instrumentalist view of the State—See Chapter 2). The goal was to wrest power from this group by struggle, struggle guided by correct class analysis. Although Jonas' writing did not delve into the issues of a vanguard group leading the struggle, cultural control, the emergence of counter groups, or into definitions of class consciousness, such elaborations were not necessary to give the overall flavor of his conflict-based argument.

The author went on to state that short-term struggles should center on increasing the supply of "building blocks" defined within the present socio-economic system. The long-term struggles should be for control of the State apparatus—a traditional conflict statement. Rather than an assuming symmetry of subsystems within a system, or of mutually reciprocal adjustments within the system, Jonas focused analysis on control of society by those with power and implications of this control for structural social change.

Rather than defining "community" in the abstract, Jonas insisted that those in the community who understood power and could organize were the ones who could struggle productively. Rather than defining groups through consensual definitions of division of labor, Jonas called up an image of class consciousness arising among persons aware of oppression and organized to attack the basic socio-economic causes of it. This consciousness might have been interpreted as an interest group consciousness, had it not been for Jonas' earlier analysis of State and market. The language and the content of his essay reflected an enthusiasm backed by optimistic expectations. The possibility for change, for far-reaching structural change both in the immediate situation and in the continuing struggle, seemed to motivate the author. The question was how to direct this change by linking theory to policy, by acknowledging the importance of both intellectual analysis and mass action.

CONFLICT THROUGH OTHER EYES

Offsetting this enthusiasm was a contradictory and somewhat more pessimistic tone in the literature. Repeated failures in implementing far-reaching community change had pushed some activists into increasingly polarized positions and had subsequently intensified in-fighting on the left. This was nowhere more clearly seen that in the failure of leftist CMHC initiatives.

The literature on the failure of the Lincoln Hospital program [13-15] clearly mirrored the contradictions between the intentions of liberal reform minded psychiatrists and the demands of working-class indigenous para-professionals. Lincoln Hospital's storefront clinics, staffed by indigenous para-professionals, were seen by traditional academics as delivering questionable care and attempting the ill-advised task of joining psychiatric care with social advocacy. These same clinics were seen by radicals as providing dead-end jobs and bandaid social control measures aimed at potential revolutionaries. Despite the eventual discontinuance of the Lincoln Hospital Program, it spawned some of the most well developed conflict analyses within the CMHC movement.

The conflict analysis developed during this period drew heavily both on orthodox class analysis and on humanist investigations into consciousness and alienation (See Chapter 2). Authors were eager to understand the limitations placed on radical change efforts, such as Lincoln Hospital, by the existing political economic arrangements. Orthodox analysts focused their attention on material reality, reflections of wealth, and power in contemporary capitalist society.

ORTHODOX ANALYSIS

Yee

Orthodox conflict analysis placed considerable emphasis on documenting classes and class factions as they impinged on CMHC operations, for example, guiding the selection of staff and patients. The argument running through this analysis was that since such of the division of labor within centers paralleled class relationships within the larger society, therapeutic work based on these distinctions could not hope to erase class-based exploitation. Centers were simply microcosms of the larger capitalist society. The cries for change, ringing in the voices of radical activists, were called forth in a developing conflict class analysis.

One of the most well developed of these analyses came out of the Lincoln Hospital experience. Published several years later by Willie Kai Yee, this research was entitled, "Dialectical Materialism and Community Mental Health: An Analysis of the Lincoln Hospital Department of Psychiatry" [16]. The adoption of traditional class analysis, wedded to dialectical materialism, distinguished this as orthodox conflict analysis. Further evidence was offered by the author's incorporation of work from orthodox conflict authors. The author began with a statement of principles of materialist dialectics from Mao, Lenin, and Engels. After an overview of the "external relations of community" for CMHC programs, including an analysis of CMHC programs as "nonproductive" and reflecting capitalist class relations, the author moved on to the internal relations of the program, including the subclasses of the Lincoln Hospital Department of Psychiatry (See Table 4).

Table 4. Subclasses in the Lincoln Hospital Department of Psychiatry

Interest Group	Job Title	Education	Income	Affiliation
Supportive workers	Housekeeper Security guard Clerk Receptionist Secretary	High school or trade school	Less than $10,000	Union 1199, or DC 37
Patient-care workers	Community mental health worker Social worker Nurse's Aide	Nursing school or some college		ANA, nurses' union
Professionals	Psychologist Resident Psychiatrist	Medical or graduate school Residency	Less than $30,000	Professional org. AMA, APA, AECOM faculty
Administrators	Unit head Dept. chairman Administrator	As above institute	Less than $50,000	Psychoanalytic institute AECOM faculty
Ruling class	Dept. chairman Member, board of trustees Dean		More than $50,000	Boards of corporation, Federation of Jewish Philanthropies

Source: Willie Kai Yee [16, p. 148].

Yee here, in typical orthodox style, was making the point that the class divisions so pervasive in the larger society were replicated within the CMHC staff, and power relationships within the staff mirrored those outside the center. Orthodox analysis stretched the view of academics who formerly concentrated on microanalysis of individual programs by enlarging their investigations to political economic formations in the larger society. In addition, the European heritage of this literature brought to its American practitioners an appreciation of class development on an international scale. Authors such as Yee were interested in class analysis within core capitalist nations, as well as alternatives presented by socialist and revolutionary nation states. The works of Marx and Mao heightened this international flavor in the American literature.

HUMANIST MARXISM: THE RADICAL COLLECTIVES

Other softer analyses in the conflict tradition had developed quite fully by the 1970s in the writing of other groups of mental health activists, for example, in the journal of the Radical Therapy collective. It was at the turn of the decade that *Radical Therapist*, a journal begun by Michael Glen, a young psychiatrist influenced by Lincoln Hospital and conflict analysis in the 1960s began to publish. Radical Therapy was based on a manifesto which read in part [17, pp. 280-282]:

1. The practice of psychiatry has been usurped by the medical establishment. Political control of its public aspects has been seized by medicine and language of soul healing (Greek term omitted here) has been infiltrated with irrelevant medical concepts and terms.
2. Extended individual psychotherapy is an elitist, outmoded, as well as non-productive form of psychiatric help. It concentrates the talents of a few on a few. It silently colludes with the notion that people's difficulties have their source within them while implying that everything is well with the world. It promotes oppression by shrouding its consequences with shame and secrecy. If further mystifies by attempting to pass as an ideal human relationship when it is, in fact, artificial in the extreme.
3. By remaining 'neutral' in an oppressive situation psychiatry, especially in the public sector, has become an enforcer of established values and laws. Adjustment to prevailing conditions is the avowed goal of most psychiatric treatment. Persons who deviate from the world's madness are given fraudulent diagnostic tests which generate diagnostic labels which lead to 'treatment' which is, in fact, a series of graded repressive procedures such as 'drug management,' hospitalization, shock therapy, perhaps lobotomy. All these forms of 'treatment' are perversions of legitimate medical methods which have been put at the service of the establishment by the medical profession. Treatment is forced on persons who would, if left alone, not seek it.

Traditional psychiatry held neither the promise of liberation from social pathology nor the technique for personal growth. From this viewpoint, community mental health could be seen chiefly as a pacification program [18]. Pacification came through cultural control. Psychiatry existed as another form of socialization to the alienation of cultural forms of capitalism. It perpetuated control rather than promoting liberation.

To this group, "community" meant a return to sharing productive labor and collective ownership of the means of that production. Overlaying this collective production would be changes in human relations. Communal living arrangements would help build a community of shared values, roles, sanctions, etc. The early Marx, the humanitarian or idealist Marx, shone through in these writings. As noted in Chapter 3, Dr. Glen began the journal while a young psychiatrist in the Air Force in North Dakota. He and a few other interested persons saw a need to focus the radical response to psychiatry through the publication of a journal. After several years of publication, he and his family moved to Boston and founded the Radical Therapy Collective. As more and more interested students, working class activists and others came to offer their views, the collective became rife with conflict itself. Eventually, Dr. Glen left and the collective members went on to other activities. Some became active in the women's movement, and others became associated with the patient's rights movement. The humanist search for non-alienated cultural styles, a search not necessarily premised on class-based revolution in the orthodox sense, drew heavily on the works of such authors as Marcuse and Fromm (see Chapter 2).

HUMANIST MARXISM: THE WEST COAST COLLECTIVE

Claude Steiner, in his edited volume *Readings in Radical Psychiatry* [19] recounts the history of the Berkeley Radical Psychiatry Center of which he was the founding father. Beginning in 1969, in the aftermath of the People's Park uprising, a Free Clinic including psychiatric services, was founded in Berkeley. Steiner along with Hogie Wyckoff and Joy Marcus, activist feminists, helped in this effort.

After a series of struggles among the leaders of the Free Clinic and among the psychiatric group, the radical psychiatry members left the administrative structure of the Free Clinic and founded an independent Radical Psychiatry Center. The Center was organized around collective living arrangements for participants and offered radical psychiatric therapy and training to new recruits. In addition to its everyday operations, the Center sponsored a well-attended conference on radical psychiatry in 1971 and several years later started publication of a journal, *Issues in Radical Therapy*. Also in 1971, the Center established offshoots in Los Angeles, San Francisco, and Sacramento.

When Michael Glenn's radical therapy group moved to Boston in 1971, the split which occurred included faction-fighting among those who considered themselves radical therapists and those who considered themselves chiefly theoreticians. The new journal published by the group, *Rough Times*, angered some of the Berkeley therapy group. This group eventually, in 1972, organized Phase II, A Berkeley Radical Psychiatry Center for group therapy.

As with the Boston group, personal and ideological infighting within the Collective ultimately resulted in its demise. By 1972 the doors to the original Center were closed. This was the result of multifaceted dissatisfaction expressed by members of the Berkeley group and voiced in an Appendix to the Steiner volume [19, pp. 187-192]. The controversy centered on new members' perceived required allegiance and deference to the original founders of the Collective. It was sensed that these founders formed a special in-group, bound together by communal living and shared relationships. This elite was seen as unduly influencing the operation of the collective. Lack of rules for entry into the Collective, lack of acceptance for legitimate criticism, and mounting hostility gradually undermined the original unity of the group. The splinter group, in their Appendix to the 1975 volume, "Resume of Criticisms," [19, pp. 187-192] voiced the feeling that members were being excluded from policy making despite the groups' elaborately articulated methods for sharing power and communicating ideas. These formal methods of communal decision making could not overcome the implicit sense of informal bonding among the originators and the sensed exclusion of new members from this privileged in-group.

In its heyday, the New Radical Psychiatry Group evolved a written *Manifesto*, also contained within the 1975 volume, espousing a blending of personal and political lives around a liberated psychiatry. The *Manifesto* was originally codified as a response to the 1969 annual conference of the American Psychiatric Association (APA) held in San Francisco. This was the famous APA conference which was disrupted by pie throwing and demonstrations by followers of radical psychiatry, gay liberation, and women's liberation.

Psychiatry, according to the Manifesto, should be nonmedical and explicitly political and liberating. "People's troubles have their source not within them but in their alienated relationships, in their exploitation, in polluted environments, in war, and in the profit motive" [19, p. 4]. Psychiatric diagnosis was mystified oppression. Personal liberation only was possible within the context of social liberation. According to Steiner, theorists who influenced this group's thinking included Marx, Laing, Marcuse and Wilhelm Reich [19, p. 143].

> Over the next four years sexism, the oppressiveness of monogamy, heterosexual and family structures, competition, the uses and abuses of power, affinity and enmity became the focus of the theory resulting in further theory about relationships, cooperation, and power.

Steiner developed a four-fold typology of psychiatrists. Alpha psychiatrists comprised the majority of medical psychiatrists and were conservative or liberal in their theory and in their therapy. Beta were conservative or liberal in their politics and radical in their therapeutic methods. Gamma psychiatrists were radical in their politics and conservative in their practice. Radical psychiatrists were those who were truly radical in both politics and psychiatric methods [19, p. 10].

Steiner fit Fritz Perls and Eric Berne into the Beta category. These he felt were truly innovative in their approach to therapy but were lacking in an alternative political ideology, an ideology which would focus their therapeutic techniques on issues of alienation and on the political roots of suffering.

Laing, and in a sense Szasz (who Steiner labeled as politically aware) were categorized as Gamma psychiatrists because of their adherence to radical politics despite their espousal of conservative therapeutic techniques such as psychoanalysis.

As part of their effort to make their psychiatry thoroughly radical, the West Coast Collective made use of such training methods as 1) Contact Raps, i.e. open discussions and self-criticism, 2) a training system based on interaction with Elders—persons who had knowledge and skill to share with learners, and 3) Peer Matching or the pairing of persons with similar interests for collective study.

Therapy was always carried out in one of two types of groups. Work Groups focused on one member at a time and employed a process of clarifying and challenging the individual over his or her stated problems. Game Groups, on the other hand, made use of a number of interactional scripts such as Rescue where one person might play the victim and others acted the roles of the rescuers. The guiding ideology underlying these group techniques was always that of overcoming the inherent sense of alienation and oppression seen as the root cause of psychiatric troubles. Pigging, or verbally attacking group members, was usually unacceptable since it was seen as heightening rather than defusing alienation. In these ways, radical theory was joined with innovative group therapy techniques.

Another work, also published by Grove Press, a press often associated with "left-wing" politics, appeared a year after the Steiner work. The volume was *Love, Therapy, and Politics: Issues in Radical Therapy-The First Year*, edited by Collective member Hogie Wyckoff [20]. This volume focused particularly on issues related to gender. It was developed despite the growing factionization within the Berkeley group and between the Boston Collective and the Berkeley group.

Although Wyckoff's approach and basic terminology are essentially those employed in the earlier work, issues of men's and women's liberation are more fully explored. Wyckoff adds articles on relations between men and women, on the use of transactional analysis in overcoming exploitative gender stereotyping, on bisexuality, and on what are characterized as varieties of oppression in society such as the normative standard of coupling one man with one woman. The volume represents a growing specialization within the overall movement toward a subspecialty dealing with women. This trend later developed into a fuller range of analyses dealing with gender authored by feminists in the tradition of the humanist marxist literature [21].

MIDDLE RANGE MARXISTS

Kunnes

In addition to these two schools of thought, the orthodox marxist and the humanist marxists, came a middle range of conflict CMHC thinkers. These writers shared a view that class conflict formed the basis of social structure and change, that values were dialectically related to class, and that legitimate power and authority in contemporary society reflected control of the ruling elite.

Several examples of this middle range conflict position found their way into important journals or CMHC volumes during the late 1960s and early 1970s. One of the most prominent examples was written by Richard Kunnes. Kunnes had been a psychiatric resident at the New York State Psychiatric Institute along with Glen, but he had dropped out and become a well-known activist in the heady days of the Lincoln Hospital strife. His style of protest against the psychiatric establishment included the pie throwing at American

Psychiatric Association conventions. By the early 1970s he had a position with the Division of Community and Social Psychiatry at Albert Einstein School of Medicine, and with the Health PAC organization. Kunnes set forth a conflict argument in an article entitled "Radicalism and Community Mental Health," published in a volume of Works, *The Critical Issues of Community Mental Health* edited by Gottesfeld in 1972 [22, pp. 35-49]. Kunnes began by presenting what he saw as the relationship between U.S. politics and psychiatry, especially community psychiatry. He approached this relationship from two assumptions: first, that the psychiatric profession was part of the U.S. sociopolitical system and second, that the system itself was the major cause of psychiatric disability.

Kunnes detailed how the psychiatric profession continued as a capitalistic enterprise. It had begun as a laissez-faire capitalism, and evolved into "the corporate liberalism of the community mental health center" [22, p. 36]. He charged that the role of the new psychiatrist was dominated by mechanisms similar to the domination of the United States economy and politics by the military industrial complex. The similarity included their emphasis on pacification and counter-insurgency. Illness and money were associated in the capitalist market. Kunnes argued that economic principles rather than psychiatric principles guided the development of community psychiatry.

This clearly was a statement within what I have called conflict tradition. The emphasis on the centrality of the capitalist economy and its manifestations in psychiatry was typical of conflict authors. The labeling of psychiatry as part of the capitalist market and in the service of the political system was likewise typical for conflict theorists in the CMHC movement, as well as the linking of consciousness to class relationships.

Kunnes went on to state that no matter what the stage of "psycho-economic evolvement we are in, psychiatry serves the system and its norms. Community mental health aims at the systematic subordination of individual behavior to false social norms" [22, pp. 36-37]. Examples of this were schools, police, roles of women, industry, the military, and psychiatrists as upholders of morals. On this last point, the author directed attention to the traditional psychiatric biases in favor of heterosexuality, male dominance, monogamy and repression of dissenters, and against acknowledgement of racism, sexism, imperialism and exploitation. This was a clear repudiation of the consensual view of the relationship between legitimate authorities and the normative value structure. For example, while the assumption by

Caplan was that psychiatrists were supporting consensual values and roles in concert with other authorities and with society as a whole, here the assumption is that psychiatrists represent simply one set of controllers, joining with other social control agents in order to uphold the culture of an elite group. As Kunnes writes [22, p. 40]

> All too often the definition of 'community psychiatry' as those programs which keep the community safe for psychiatry has become the reality of community mental health programs.

Rather than enhancing the conditions for change, such programs prevented it; they served as pacification programs, as programs promoting law and order. By focusing concern on issues of mental health and away from "efforts to confront the basic oppressive institution in our society," [22, p. 42] these programs maintained the establishment's *status quo*. They depoliticized issues, "psychiatricizing" them instead.

The correct analysis of the community in community mental health, according to Kunnes, rested on conceptualizing [22, p. 43]

> community control . . . in its broadest sense, namely that in which a community itself controls and determines the political, social, and economic realities of the community. We cannot talk about community mental health without a community and we cannot talk about a community until it has a political consciousness of itself and is self-controlled.

Such control should extend to elected boards from the community directing decisions about treatment, funding, research and education. Those who promoted professionalism, instead of promoting artificial hierarchies, could simplify the division of labor and base it on expertise and community need. Theory and practice, in Kunnes' vision, must come from the masses and must serve a politically viable group. Theory should no longer be a perpetuation of elitist knowledge by persons trained in elite institutions. In a sense, Kunnes was suggesting the development of the American equivalent of the Chinese barefoot doctor—a peasant with specialized medical skills who worked half a day as a peasant laborer and the other half as a doctor. Kunne seemed to envision a kind of barefoot psychiatrist who would be chosen to serve the people as one of them rather than being chosen from among the dominant elite to foster social control on the masses.

But what of the catchment concept? According to Kunnes, the concept itself was laudatory if used to end exclusionary services policies. But [22, p. 47],

> In practical terms, institutional opposition to catchment areas arises from the vision of community controlled funding, planning, and administration for entire areas. Imperialistically oriented professionals shrink from the day, which is rapidly approaching, where a 'lay' board of catchment area residents will write contracts for services from professional institutions and then will evaluate the services rendered.

Clearly, Kunnes was inspired by a vision of conflict and change, by the prophetic call to an equalitarian social order and humanitarian respect for need-based services. What differentiated him so clearly from the orthodox conflict analysts was his lack of firm class analysis, critical assessments of market processes, and detailed analysis of what orthodox authors would have called the external relations of production as mirrored in capitalist social relations. Kunnes' marxism, however distasteful to his orthodox colleagues, linked him much more closely to the conflict tradition than to the consensual.

There was no question but that Kunnes rejected a systems or field approach to social analysis. He did not think that a population could be objectively carved into catchment areas regardless of ideologies and called a community. Nor did he think that contemporary populations could exist under a grand consensus of culture without domination of the capitalist elite. To Kunnes, legitimate authorities were not representing the will of the people, nor were academics simply plying their scientific insights for the good of all. His break with consensualism was complete, as was that of conflict scholars in general. They had overtly adopted the rhetoric of conflict analysis and thereby raised a myriad of questions ignored within the earlier consensual literature.

Cross national comparisons of these years show the broader context in which such issues were addressed. The best overview being perhaps Peter Sedgwick's review of anti-psychiatry literature and what he termed Psycho Politics [23]. Sedgwick traced the rise in Britain, Italy, and France of a European marxist critique of psychiatry. Moving beyond the concept of post-World War II therapeutic communities, activists in Italy in the late 1960s turned to the development of "mental health politics based on neighborhood collectives and anti-hierarchical work teams (which) gathered a particular momentum from the communitarian politics fostered by 'May events' of 1968 in France and their sequel in Italy over 1968-69" [23, p. 209]. A particularly interesting contrast case from cross national psychiatry involves events in the People's Republic of China—a case much discussed in the American psychiatric literature during the 1970s.

SOCIALISM AND THE THEORY OF MENTAL ILLNESS: THE CASE OF P.R.C.

A host of American psychiatrists and other mental health workers travelled to the People's Republic of China (P.R.C.) after the re-establishment of political relations in the early 1970s. They returned to publish numerous descriptive reports about psychiatric treatment facilities which they had toured. This surge of interest in what was a self-proclaimed Marxist system of treatment swept through the American mental health literature [24-26]. Such fascination with the Chinese approach lent an aire of legitimacy to homegrown conflict theorists within the mental health literature and therefore deserves special attention here.

China, in the early part of the 20th century, had been plagued with massive mental and social pathology including alcoholism, drug addiction, psychosis, criminal behavior, prostitution, and a host of other clusters of behaviors termed deviant [27, p. 415]. Marxism, developed in the Maoist tradition, defined these as reflections of the dominant mode of production, i.e. capitalism, and China's legacy of imperialism. The overwhelming powerlessness of the masses of Chinese was evident not only in poverty and physical disease, but in the cultural, social, political and economic structures which directed their lives. Deviance from these, whether acted out in withdrawal through addiction, psychosis, or criminal behavior represented a common political act under the Maoist ideology.

Visiting scholars and professionals in the 1970s were taught that after the Communist Revolution in 1949, amelioration of deviance was tied to political reform. These reforms took the shape of complex cycles of infrastructure change such as land reform, experimentation with national monetary and fiscal policies, with urban and rural industrialization, with population movements for communalization, and with programs of material and ideology work incentives. Such reforms were aimed at creating not only an emerging communal economy but a communal consciousness [28]. Health reforms, including mental health reforms, were built into every level of this revolution. Since disease was defined as a class enemy much like any other "remnant from the bitter past," political mass movement strategy was defined as "treatment" [29].

The Chinese rejected the idea that Maoist views of society were separate from the Marxist-Leninist tradition. Nonetheless, Mao's essays on philosophy did amend and extend some of the earlier marxist works on perception and cognition. Marx and Lenin, for example, had written on the relationship between external reality and internal mental activity, later expanded by Pavlovian behaviorism. Mao, in his essay, "On Practice" written in 1937, set forth the marxist answer to: How do we know? [30]. He wrote that knowing is based on two stages of cognition, phenomenal plus judgement and inference through practice. Knowing, he emphasized, is based on a dialectical materialist process, and evolves through social practice. Social practice (action in the world) alters the reality of things and also perceptions. This dialectical process is continual and evolving. It is summed up in his phrase, practice-knowledge-practice. He wrote that if you want to know the taste of a pear, you must change the pear by eating it yourself. If you want to know revolution, you must participate in it yourself.

Mao wrote that the existence of one reality creates possibilities for internal contradictions and the emergence of opposites. For example, if the State imprisons persons for political views, the very gathering together of these persons creates the potential for unity and action against the imprisonment.

Mao stressed that any event must be interpreted in its social context and analyzed within this dialectical process of change. Such analysis leads to an appreciation of perceptions of varied realities. He also discussed criticism and self-criticism, setting forth the basic path to handling contradictions within the people [30, p. 345].

> The law of contradiction in things, that is, the law of the unity of opposites, is the fundamental law of nature and of society and therefore also the fundamental law of thought. It stands opposed to the metaphysical world outlook. It represents a great revolution in the history of human knowledge. According to dialectal materialism, contradiction is present in all processes of objectively existing things and of subjective thought and permeates all these processes from beginning to end; this is the universality and absoluteness of contradiction. Each contradiction and each of its aspects have their respective characteristics; this is the particularity and relativity of contradiction.

Contradiction is universal, implicit in historical reality, and in the perception of that reality. This evolving dialectic directs contradictions which cannot be concretized or frozen in time. Entities that exist in one form, in one context today, may be quite changed tomorrow.

This and other essays exhorted persons to re-evaluate interpersonal interactions and their own consciousness. Criticism and self-criticism were practiced in small groups throughout the country, and structured into on-going study groups at the neighborhood level. In 1958, Mao issued his four principles for health: serve workers, peasants and soldiers; regard prevention as the principal activity; unite Western and Chinese traditional doctors; and combine public health with mass movements. Under the direction of these principles, and later during the Cultural Revolution's barefoot doctor program [31, p. 7021] mental health was integrated at every level of the Chinese health system. At the lowest organization level, Chinese rural barefoot doctors or urban red medical workers counseled troubled individuals and provided major and minor tranquilizers. At central levels, more highly trained personnel and physicians with psychiatric training treated in-patients in general or mental hospitals.

One interesting example of the application of Maoist principles to mental health policy is reviewed in Yi-Huang Lu's article, "The Collective Approach to Psychiatric Practice in the People's Republic of China" [32]. In this work, the impact of collective responsibility in psychiatric treatment and in hospital administration and policy are explored. The importance of the principle, 'serve the people,' is investigated as it relates to actual therapy, as well as the minimalization of elitism among workers in the hospital, and finally, the revolutionary optimism that pervades treatment and social experience in general.

In such a case as the People's Republic of China, it is relatively easy to explore the connection between conflict theory and political action. The persona of Mao was constructed to reflect a real and metaphorical conjuncture of conflict theory with State policy relating to mental health and every other aspect of Chinese life.

CONSENSUS RETRENCHES

One should never wear one's best trousers to go out and battle for freedom and truth [33].

In the United States not only had conflict theorists developed their rhetoric within an international arena, but consensualists were finding it harder than ever to ignore even the mildest of humanist conflict critiques. Liberal reformers, after all, formed the core of academic psychiatrists justifying the CMHC movement to the public and the legislature. They, too, now were getting their trousers dirty in confrontations. Caplan was not alone in facing angry blacks across tables during community consultations.

The reaction of leaders of the CMHC movement, the academics and administrators to pressures from the mass movements on the streets, and also from lower level workers within the movement, was at least twofold: 1) a growing trend toward modifying legislation and regulations to increase mandated services and target them to special populations such as the elderly, youth, and drug addicts; and 2) an increase in attempts to analyze services with an eye toward controlling them.

The first point, the targeting of special populations, was reflected in the 1970 hearings. Special notice was taken of disadvantaged areas, with seed monies going to active community groups. The defining of target populations was seen both as the answer to militant demands for services and as a way to pin down the meaning of "community" for evaluation.

Avoiding systematic models of class interests or historically based class factions, the best targets academics could define were collections of immediately identifiable special interests, including drug addicts, who had been attracting attention since addicted veterans had been returning from Vietnam. In addition there were children, ethnic minorities, and the generic "disadvantaged."

For the CMHC literature, this meant that a hodgepodge of special interests were thrust forward as populations in "the community." Grunebaum, in his *The Practice of Community Mental Health* covered the field in a typical way by including mention of children, adolescents, the family, the mentally retarded, the subnormal, the corrections system, the alcoholic, the poor, the drug addicts, and the geriatric patient [34]. From a sociological standpoint, such collectivities could hardly be considered representative of the broader social structure or even of culturally related groups.

The consensual systems model, however, allowed authors great leeway in defining such groups. Since all groups were in some way integrated into the larger system or field, sharing the larger "community" consensus, their functioning could be interpreted simply in relationship to this larger system. Were the target groups receiving their equitable amount of services? Were they being adequately represented in the governing of centers? Were they being excluded because of costs or cultural barriers? Such administrative questions began to occupy the writings of the times and fueled the fires of evaluation research. Social indices of community based on census data were developed by National Institute of Mental Health (NIMH), and attention began turning to "scientific" analyses of needs and services for these social groups [35].

How were consensualists to respond to the persistent presence of conflict on the streets and at their doors, while also acknowledging the legitimacy of their own work? The "interest group" route was one answer. By acknowledging the demands of such groups, but insisting on expansion of traditional services to them for their problems, consensualist's could serve both liberal reformist and expansion of the psychiatric market.

COMMUNITY AS FRANCHISER

Panzetta

An important example of this strategy was written in 1971 by Anthony F. Panzetta [36], a Philadelphia psychiatrist. In "The Concept of Community: The Short Circuit of the Mental Health Movement," Panzetta suggested that the catchmenting of services resulted in those services having to react to highly visible phenomena in their geographic areas. One alternative to this artificial focusing of action was to conceptualize community as a dimension of time, a community of shared experiences, or what I have called a non-class based special interest group. Panzetta's answer to how a CMHC should relate to its community was to identify itself to the area and to include in its decision making persons residing in that area. Such people had to be interested in the center, able to conceptualize problems and solutions, and willing to participate in center affairs.

Panzetta's essay was neither as clearly consensual as Caplan's nor as clearly conflictual as Glen's. It represented a consensual interest group model of community, and rested on a consensual view of community as interest groups. Issues related to power and authority, as well as issues of change and revolution, clearly were salient to the author. Panzetta's model of relationships between centers and their communities was based on analysis of power relationships, not on assumed consensual norms or integrated systems. But Panzetta suggested that consumers simply relate to centers through the given market system. Clients should use the center if they liked it, or stay away if they didn't. Beyond this, the center staff decided who was able to control policy and practice. The fact that center personnel might be quite elitist as far as race or class or sex and quite unlike their clients with respect to these features, was glossed over by the author. He seemed to assume that professionals were trained to serve regardless of the setting. Panzetta had no concern with structural, political-economic change, only with the development of interest groups. His interest group model could not explain or predict the emergence and importance of one special interest group over another. Collective conflict was not seen as emergent from class conflict but as a residue of interest group oppression. Nonetheless, power and conflict were addressed more directly than they had been in the writings of other consensualists. Just how directly they were addressed could be seen in another work the same year by Panzetta, 1971, a book entitled, *Community Mental Health: Myth and Reality*. The front piece of this work clearly reflected the author's concern over issues of power and conflict, a concern equally salient to others in the CMHC movement. It pictured, among many amusing but powerful symbols, a tortuous pathway for CMHC ideas, running through a myth machine, past the dragons of white and black power, past the time bomb of local control, past the budget cutting of state control, and finally ending up in the sewer system. The dragons of white and black power did indeed breath fire on the CMHC movement, heating up its theory and practice. Advocates of community control threw bombs, and bureaucrats lay in wait at every turn.

Although Panzetta's concept of community as "franchiser" for centers might have carried intellectual appeal, it did little to guide the basic changes efforts of militant groups. The suggestion that a community could simply refuse to buy the services of a center, thereby making community displeasure known, was certainly not a solution to the activists who saw such services as monopolies of professionals and corporate interests franchised by the federal government.

Centers continued to be confronted with demands, and their administrators' responses were as angry and as militant in support of their services as were the criticisms of the so-called "community" militants. In fact, hostility in public meetings was in some cases more clearly demonstrated by "legitimate authorities" than by the outside "militants" [37].

COMMUNITY AS CONSENSUS

Rhodes

The centers were being caught in a squeeze. Nixon, firmly entrenched by 1971, began cutting CMHC funds. The economy was sagging and the legislature heard new calls for accountability. Anger over issues of power and control was voiced not only in the writings of the conflict theorists but in consensual interest group literature as well. How did the mainstream react? One answer is found in the *Handbook of Community Mental Health*, a massive tome published in 1972 and edited by Golann and Eisdorfer [38]. One of the most influential volumes of its kind, it consisted of more than 1000 pages, and covered a wide spectrum of theoretical and practical topics on the movement.

Issues of power and conflict were central to the introductory essay by the editors. Everett Hughes was quoted by the authors as supporting the legitimacy of professional control and this quotation was juxtaposed with an anti-professionalism statement by a radical therapist. The editors wrote [38, p. 14]:

> The major issue of the 1960s has been the achievement of increased flexibility and comprehensiveness of mental health services. The major issue of the 1970s will be that of community control over the mental health field, a process that to date has largely been initiated by professionals and taken by the urban poor.

Clearly dragons' breath had been felt throughout the movement.

Despite this, the consensual systems model, as reflected in this volume, had hardly sustained a dent. The very first section of the volume was entitled, "Community Systems and Behavior"—systems were clearly alive and well. In addition, there were sections on education as a humanizing vehicle (an emphasis closely akin to Caplan's view of change through understanding and communication); a study of the health "system" as it is characterized by a "dynamic equilibrium" a phrase often used in consensual models of structure and function; and works on a variety of legitimate authorities and their relationship to the movement, including selections dealing with the criminal justice system, religious systems, welfare systems, and military communities. The first major article in the volume was perhaps the most telling in terms of the new polarization of the consensual model.

The first article, "Regulation of Community Behavior: Dynamics and Structure," was written by William C. Rhodes Professor of Psychology and of Community Health at the University of Michigan [39]. Dr. Rhodes presented a view of community taken from animal etiology, a model based on an excitor-reactor exchange whereby a community reacted toward deviance in ways similar to animals reacting to unusual situations or deviants in their midst. Depending on the "mood" of the community, a variety of systems could be called into action to confront the deviance. These systems ranged from police, courts, and detention to more sympathetic modes of response including education, welfare, and mental health.

The community power structure acted as a mediator between the community will and deviance. An overall behavior regulatory system was composed of organization components with missions mandated by the government. Their structure was composed of a consensually agreed upon ideational construct of behavior, an associated body of knowledge, a professional apparatus, a set of professional legitimate authorities, a training structure for the guilds, sets of sanctions for behavior, and "a set of hallmark behavior regulating operational patterns through which all of these elements are discharged into the community and brought to bear upon human behavior" [39, pp. 25-26].

Rhodes explained the operation of each of these and the operational patterns and systems in terms of behavior construction, deterrence, and reconstruction. He stressed the historical importance of the family and religion in regulating behavior, but he suggested that their importance had diminished in the face of growing humanism and charities. With this change came the organization of professional guilds and the use of scientific knowledge. Guilds became associated with the government and played an increasing role in community life.

This was a thoroughly consensual analysis of the growth of social control. Religion and family were seen as evolved socializing subsystems supporting individuals and socializing them to the community consensus. Rhodes did not take the analysis a step further to talk about the relationship between these institutions and potential repression in the service of the State. There was no mention of differing definitions of normative behavior by class; this was to come in his more developed work.

The author devoted the last several pages to his analysis to the "winds of change." He noted that population pressures had produced growth and shifts in community. Also of paramount importance were changes in the relationships between the mainstream culture bearers and the negatively sanctioned population. This relationship, which for so long had been stable, was now becoming fluid. While formerly the mainstream had been able to define what was deviant, the deviants were now insisting on their legitimate right to fulfill new roles, to establish new intergroup relationships. "They are insisting upon a new relationship between themselves and the mainstream culture bearers (as seen, for instance in the Negro population)" [39, p. 33]. This was being manifested in such groups as welfare recipient, Puerto Ricans, homosexuals, and drug addicts.

This rebelliousness was based on two beliefs: that the theoretically "uncomplicated culture bearers and culture enforcers are actually deeply implicated in the sources of community stress," and that "the dominant culture bearing group deliberately creates, maintains, and supports the conditions which make it possible to label them in negative ways" [39, p. 33].

Rhodes' discussion was one of the fullest descriptions of the consensual model. The dichotomy he drew between the mainstream and the outsiders was boldly set forth despite the recognition of the diversity among the non-dominant groups. This latter group included ethnic groups, groups based on sexual preference, and groups identified through their economic standing. With one sweep of his consensual brush, they all were painted as deviants.

Why were such conflicts now addressed by even the most conservative of authors? The answer comes from analysis of the political economic times. The market expansion had brought the federal government into the funding of direct services and had financed the entrance of large numbers of competitive sector employees in the mental illness treatment system. The services had also served the State by expanding the infrastructure for both public and private sectors of the capitalist market, and had put in place the services from which the monopoly sector professionals and corporate interests could make their profits. In addition, these services had carried with them a form of social control which touched diverse sectors of the population. Such cultural control could be balanced off against overt control by the State apparatus.

It was clear that in such times of unrest, change could not be ignored even by the most insulated of intellectuals. The strain showed in the most conservative of priestly writings. The consensualists were themselves conflicted. The fact that interest groups were considered to be change agents instead of just deviants was telling. Conflict theorists tied such movements to historical forces directing class consciousness and change; consensual theorists viewed them as time-limited manifestations of socio-cultural dysfunctions.

Dr. Rhodes presented an extended version of the same conceptual model in his work *Behavioral Threat and Community Response: A Community Psychology Inquiry*, also published in 1972 [40]. In this work he spelled out in detail what he termed the "threat-recoil" process consisting of behaviors by individuals or collectivities which threaten the majority community. The process begins with an activator which challenges the community culture bearers. Such an activator could consist of drugs, sexual deviation, mental illness, etc. [40, p. 11]. Social agencies are seen as taking an active role in defining the threat to the community, and they might be called upon by varying power structures (such as judicial or legislative bodies) to form alliances against the threat [40, p. 21]. Professionals function as community protectors. The power structure plays the role of arbiter "of judgement and accommodation" between the threatening sector and the majority culture [40, p. 27].

In this book, Dr. Rhodes pictured community in a more dynamic and fragmented state than seemed to have been the case in his article. He acknowledged that there is "a more or less constant steady state of uneasiness in the community" arising from the ongoing threats [40, p. 10]. This realization is woven throughout the book, backed by citations from Marcuse and supported in statements in the Postscript which refer to the voices of discontent which echoed all around the author, in the United States and throughout the world.

Another interesting aspect of this work is Dr. Rhodes' acknowledgment of the relationship between socio-economic class and the threat cycle. As with most priestly works, class is not the Marxian class as defined through relations to the means of production. Class is assumed to be related to income, wealth, education, etc.—a priestly approach to class. Nonetheless, Dr. Rhodes cites the connections between the lower socio-economic class and the propensity to be in the minority-agitator group. Such conditions as higher psychological distress and one parent families (referred to as pseudo families, jerry-built facsimiles of modal family units in American communities [40, p. 33]) are seen as being potential sources of threat. Disorganized area of sites, are seen as potential cites of threats, as the author writes [40, p. 37]:

> In the United States, such neighborhoods are the semi-permanent habitat for specially culturally stagnant groups such as Negroes, Mexicans and Puerto Ricans.

These neighborhoods are identified as being the breeding ground for vice, psychopathology, and other sources of deviance. The responder group is more frequently from the middle class and bearers of the Protestant-Christian-Judaic ethic [40, p. 39].

Despite this extremely conservative consensual approach, the author does write of the sweeping changes which cultural doctrines and social institutions are undergoing. He feels that the "whole infrastructure of behavior regulation is involved in this eruption of change" [40, p. 100]. Both the community and the individual will have to adapt to the new sense of strangeness which these increasingly frequent threats are posing. As Rhodes states, "The strangeness is awesome and bewildering to us" [40, p. 107]. Regulatory machinery is seen as necessarily adjusting to these conditions and attaining a new and better flexibility. In the end, Rhodes reaches the conclusion that responders must look not only to controlling the undesirable aspects of those making the threats, but to [40, p. 122]:

> . . . freeing the culture bearer from tyrannizing the demeaning aspects of his own culture, particularly from those harsh aspects that cause him to be overbearing and depressive toward his inner nature and toward those who depart from cultural repressions.

Indeed, Dr. Rhodes represented a case where the most conservative of consensual priests moved to adjust to the outpouring of prophetic argument.

COMMUNITY AS ECOLOGICAL FIELD

Two other interesting approaches to community which emerged from community psychology in the mid to late 1960s were dynamic adaptations of ecological models from biology and fluid consensual models from the social sciences. The first of these was reflected in an article by Kelly, "Toward an Ecological Conception of Preventive Interventions" [41]. Dr. Kelly was a professor of clinical psychology and presented his model in several talks and papers in the 1960s and 1970s [42, 43]. His model of the social environment was drawn from field biology and relied heavily upon concepts of interdependency and reciprocity between structures and functions. Unlike the earlier Parsonian structural-functionalism, this approach was highly dynamic, emphasizing the succession of groups in a given social environment. The idea was that, like simpler biological organism, humans to some extent used up a nitch in the environment until they were succeeded by another group who existed in a state of equilibrium in that new environment. Dr. Kelly transferred this approach to understanding coping styles in male high school students. While not leaving the priestly school of theorists, such social ecologist brought a greatly enhanced sense of change to the consensual model. Their organicism lent a perspective of continuing growth and change to the earlier priestly perspective.

A similar sense of ongoing change within the priestly model was imparted by Glidewell [44]. An educational psychologist, Dr. Glidewell emphasized the need of community mental health workers to look beyond the temporary therapeutic dyad to the possibility of change within the larger society. He wrote of the injustices and inequalities to which certain groups in the society were subject, and he asked the questions whether psychologists or to others knew how to change society, and if such changes would be for the better? In telling passage, the author wrote [44, p. 107],

> The great injustice of society is not that the lower classes have fewer resources; it is that the lower classes do not know how to get back from the system an equitable return for what they put into it.

It would seem that the implicit assumption here was that equitable returns were in fact possible, even if they were not the norm for all groups.

REFERENCES

1. M. Deutcher and M. R. Green, Mental Health Is a Social Problem, *American Journal of Orthopsychiatry*, *37*, pp. 832-834, 1967.
2. L. J. Duhl and R. L. Leopold (eds.), *Mental Health and Urban Social Policy*, Jossey-Bass, Inc., San Francisco, pp. 16-19, 1969.
3. H. S. Hughes, Emotional Disturbance and American Social Change: 1944-1969, *American Journal of Psychiatry*, *126*, pp. 21-28, 1969.
4. D. Colfax and J. Roach (eds.), *Radical Sociology*, Basic Books, New York, 1971.
5. V. Navarro, Work Ideology and Science: The Case of Medicine, *International Journal of Health Services*, *10*, pp. 523-549, 1980.
6. H. B. Waitzkin and B. Waterman, *The Exploitation of Illness in Capitalist Society*, Bobbs-Merrill, Indianapolis, 1974.
7. Health Policy Action Committee, *Mental Health for the Masses*, Health PAC, New York, May, 1969.
8. S. Dinitz and N. Beran, Community Mental Health as a Boundaryless and Boundary-Busting System, *Journal of Health and Social Behavior*, *12*, pp. 99-108, 1971.

9. H. W. Dunham, *Social Realities and Community Psychiatry*, Behavioral Publications, New York, 1976.
10. R. W. Friedrichs, *A Sociology of Sociology*, Basic Books, New York, 1970.
11. S. Kahn, *How People Get Power*, McGraw Hill, New York, 1970.
12. S. Jonas, A Theoretical Approach to the Question of Community Control of Health Services Facilities, *American Journal of Public Health*, *61*:5, pp. 916-921, 1971.
13. R. Kaplan and M. Roman, *The Organization and Delivery of Mental Health Services in the Ghetto: The Lincoln Hospital Experience*, Prager Press, New York, 1973.
14. E. Hallowitz and F. Reissman, The Role of the Indigenous Non-professional in a Community Mental Health Neighborhood Service Center Program, *American Journal of Orthopsychiatry*, *37*, pp. 766-778, 1967.
15. M. Roman, Community Control and the Community Mental Health Center: A View from Lincoln Bridge, in *Community Mental Health: Social Action and Reaction.*, B. Denner and R. Price (eds.), Holt, Rinehardt and Winston, New York, pp. 270-284, 1969.
16. W. K. Yee, Dialectical Materialism and Community Mental Health Programs: An Analysis of the Lincoln Hospital Department of Psychiatry, in *Topias and Utopias In Health*, S. Ingman and A. Thomas (eds.), Aldine Publishers, Chicago, pp. 141-158, 1975.
17. J. Agel, *The Radical Therapist Collective*, Balantine Books, New York, 1971.
18. J. Statman, Community Mental Health as a Pacification Program, *The Radical Therapist*, *1*, pp. 14-15, 1970.
19. C. Steiner, H. Wyckoff, D. Goldstine, P. Lariviere, R. Schwebel, J. Marcus, and Members of the Radical Psychiatry Center (eds.), *Readings in Radical Psychiatry*, Grove Press, New York, 1975.
20. H. Wyckoff (ed.), *Love, Therapy and Politics: Issues in Radical Therapy—The First Year*, Grove Press, New York, 1976.
21. The Socialist Feminist Commission of the New American Movement, *Women Organizing: A Socialist Feminist Bulletin*, The New American Movement, Chicago, 1979.
22. R. Kunnes, Radicalism and Community Mental Health, in *The Critical Issues in Community Mental Health*, H. Gottsfeld (ed.), Behavioral Publishers, New York, 1972.
23. P. Sedgwick, *Psycho Politics*, Harper & Row, New York, 1982.
24. S. Akhtar, *Health Care in the People's Republic of China: A Bibliography with Abstracts*, IDRC-038e, Ottawa, Canada, 1978.
25. V. W. Sidel and R. Sidel, *Serve the People: Observations on Medicine in the People's Republic of China*, Josiah Macy, Jr. Foundation, New York, 1973.
26. J. C. Cheng, Psychiatry in Traditional Chinese Medicine, *Canadian Psychiatric Association Journal*, *15*, pp. 399-401, 1970.
27. C. C. Seldon, Conditions in South China in Relation to Insanity, *American Journal of Psychiatry*, *70*, 1910.

28. J. Horn, Away with All Pests, *Monthly Review of Books*, New York, 1969.
29. R. Sidel, The Role of Revolutionary Optimism in the Treatment of Mental Illness in the P.R.C., *American Journal of Orthopsychiatry, 43*, pp. 732-736, 1973.
30. M. Tse-Tung, On Practice, in *Selected Works of Mao Tse-Tung*, Vol. I., Peking, Foreign Language Press, pp. 295-309, 1967.
31. R. K. M. New, Barefoot Doctors and Health Care in China, *Eastern Horizon*, 1974.
32. Y-C. Lu, The Collective Approach to Psychiatric Practice in the People's Republic of China, *Social Problems, 26*, pp. 2-14, 1978.
33. American Psychiatric Association, *Task Force on Community Issues in Community Psychology and Preventive Mental Health*, Behavioral Publications, New York, 1971.
34. H. Grunebaum (ed.), *The Practice of Community Mental Health*, Little, Brown & Company, Boston, 1970.
35. A. J. Kahn, *Theory and Practice of Social Planning*, Russell Sage Foundation, New York, 1969.
36. A. F. Panzetta, The Concept of Community: The Short-Circuit of the Mental Health Movement, *Archives of General Psychiatry, 25*, pp. 291-297, 1971.
37. M. L. Moore, The Role of Hostility and Militancy in Indigenous Community Health Advisory Groups, *American Journal of Public Health, 61*, pp. 922-930, 1971.
38. S. E. Golann and C. Eisdorfer (eds.), *Handbook of Community Mental Health*, Appleton-Century-Croft, New York, 1972.
39. W. C. Rhodes, Regulation of Community Behavior: Dynamics and Structure, in *Handbook of Community Mental Health*, S. Golann and C. Eisdorfer (eds.), Apple-Century-Croft, New York, 1972.
40. W. C. Rhodes, *Behavioral Threat and Community Response: A Community Psychology Inquiry*, Behavioral Publications, New York, 1972.
41. J. G. Kelly, Toward an Ecological Conception of Preventive Intervention, in *Research Contributions from Psychology to Community Mental Health*, J. W. Carter (ed.), Behavioral Publishers, New York, pp. 75-99, 1968.
42. J. G. Kelly, Ecological Constraints on Mental Health Services, *American Psychologist, 21*, pp. 535-539, 1966.
43. J. G. Kelly, Social and Community Interventions, *Annual Review of Psychology, 28*, pp. 323-361, 1977.
44. J. C. Glidewell, New Psychosocial Competence, Social Change, and Tension Management, in *Research Contributions from Psychology to Community Mental Health*, J. W. Carter (ed.), Behavioral Publications, New York, pp. 100-110, 1968.

CHAPTER 7

Theory in Phase Three with Quiescence of Conflict the Early 1970s to 1980, Aftermath from 1980 to 1990

If the 1960s could be called the era of conflict, the 1970s could be called the era of accountability. Accountability became the watchword for the CMHC movement as a whole. Programs had to be accountable to the federal government for their finances; to patients, communities and to special interests for quality and quantity [1, 2]. The earlier CMHC coalition tying together key federal legislators, federal administrators, and powerful figures in psychiatry fragmented in the late 1960s. This left the CMHC movement much more susceptible to influence by the executive branch, which was by 1972 firmly under the control of President Nixon and his allies. With the slowing of the economy, the Nixon administration lost little time in cutting the flow of monies to the program and insisting on new evidence of its worth.

The demonstrations and angry rhetoric, which had given so much impetus to radical theorists in the previous decade, faded from view. No longer were anti-establishment radicals so visible in the quest, and the influence of this loss on both the writings and the organization of CMHC activists was pronounced.

Social theorists still criticized traditional consensual social psychiatry, but did so from a non-class based, non-conflict oriented point of view. The angry young community organizers of the previous decade were absorbed into less visible programmatic change efforts or were "controlled" in any of a number of ways. Gone from the mainstream literature was the language of dialectical analyses of historical inequality, or even language which vaguely hinted at former conflict humanist alternatives. In their place were Ralph Nader-style consumer groups based on middle-class liberal critiques of psychiatry.

LEGISLATION: A LEGACY OF SPECIAL INTERESTS

The decade of the 1970s began with attempts by CMHC personnel and politicians to define a host of special client-interest groups for inclusion in services. Until this time, amendments to the legislation had mentioned the need to deliver services to consumer groups but had left the definition of consumers rather general. The 1972 regulations stated that each state mental health plan was to rank catchment areas in terms of percentage of families in the catchment with income at or below poverty level as designated by national standards. According to the new federal regulations [3] those with 25 percent of families below this poverty standard were to be designated as poverty areas. Areas so designated could apply to the Department of Health, Education and Welfare, (HEW), (later to become the separate Department of Education and the Department of Health and Human Services), for poverty designation if [3, p. 4]:

> (1) At least one-half of the population of such areas had one or more impoverished sub-areas; (2) the percentage of families with incomes below the poverty level . . . who live in such impoverished sub-areas is at least one and a half times greater than the percentage of families with incomes below the poverty level living in the least poor of the areas of that state initially designated as poverty areas . . .; (3) the project, facility or program of services for which the applicant seeks support does or will focus on the needs of such impoverished sub-areas.

As the Ralph Nader-lead group on mental health [4] was to report several years later, these changes meant that now more than 50 percent of the existing centers could be labeled as being in poverty areas. This definitional slight-of-hand occurred shortly after a Government Accounting Office (GAO) report charging, among other things, that centers were not adequately being targeted for poverty areas.

By mid-decade, however, the Ford Administration had taken over and the CMHC legislation, after being vetoed at the last minute in

1974, and vetoed again in 1975, was finally passed when Congress overrode the veto. The old coalition of Congressional leaders backing the original legislation, including Claiborne Pell and Lister Hill, had lost their small network of influentials on the federal level. They found that the decade of the 1960s had brought with it hosts of new lobbyists and increasingly polarized view on the centers' program. No longer were a rather small group of legislators and bureaucrats in CMHC in control of the program. Opinion had split not only between the executive branch and the legislature, but between factions of the legislative branch itself. Ironically, the administration at this juncture objected to the expenditure of federal funding for what it now saw as too narrowly defined a program. The administration charged the program "would not be consistent with the development of an integrated, flexible, health-service delivery system" [5, p. 54]. These new narrowly defined services which were added to the former five mandatory services included services for children and elderly, and consultation and education to such groups as health professionals, schools, courts, state and local law enforcement and correctional agencies, clergy, public welfare agencies, and health services delivery agencies. In addition, further stipulations were included to direct that services be interconnected and accessible to ethnic groups, poverty groups, and consumer groups, who were not required to be involved in policy formation [5, p. 55].

This elaboration of special interests filtered down from the general theoretical literature into the non-theoretical writings of administrators and planners. It permeated the movement as a whole.

The impact of this drive for accountability and the accompanying elaboration of interest groups will here be traced through several separate but related aspects of the CMHC literature. First, the writing of theorists will be discussed; next, middle range theorists of the movement who concentrated on interest group approaches will be reviewed, and, along with them, their compatriots in consultation and evaluation research. Throughout this analysis the question will be asked how such works reflected or failed to reflect conflict and consensus sociology.

PURE THEORY: CRITIQUE WITHOUT CLASS

Although general theoretical statements within the CMHC movement had never been numerous, their frequency declined dramatically in the 1970s. As Lounsbury et al. showed in their 1979 content analysis of the *Community Mental Health Journal*, in that one journal, general definitional works and think pieces declined steadily from 12.1 percent of all articles in 1965-1968, to 11.6 percent in 1969-1972, and then dropped again to 8.5 percent in 1973-1976 [6, p. 272]. In the literature, less and less attention was paid to social theoretical analyses. The polarization of models in the 1960s was short lived. Authors whose works were given wide circulation no longer seemed concerned with reacting to societal class conflict or its rhetoric in the impassioned tone of the 1960s.

Example of this quieter theoretical tone are seen in the works of James D. Preston on field theory, Warren Dunham on social theory and the CMHC movement, and an exchange of theoretical views on community control in response to writings by Alberta Nassi.

Preston

Preston's work was important not only for its content but also for its context. It appeared as the sole sociologic essay on community contained in the first book which was devoted totally to social science critiques of the CMHC movement. This volume, *Social Perspectives on Community Mental Health* [7] published in 1974, was produced by and for the Society for the Study of Social Problems, a reform-minded activist group of social scientists. As the editors of the volume, Roman and Trice, wrote in the introduction of their work, the Society is interested in applying expertise to "real-world issues of modern society" [7, p. vii]. It was clear that these editors were not bent on supporting or apologizing for professional psychiatry or the CMHC movement. They wrote that "the movement is at the point where analysis must replace paeans," [7, p. 2] and that, rather than representing psychiatry's third revolution, as Bellak had earlier pronounced, the movement more clearly represented psychiatry's "first proliferation"—hardly a conciliatory assessment.

Despite these harsh words, the essay which these editors chose to include in their volume, an essay on theory of the community by James Preston, was firmly rooted in consensual thought.

In his *The Meaning of 'Community' in Community Psychiatry*, [8] Dr. Preston, first, reviewed a number of traditional sociological approaches to the concept of community including ecological approaches such as zonal theory; the social system perspective, heavily premised on the work of Parsons; cultural-ethnographic approaches, such as anthropological studies of small towns; monographs using the community as a convenient research site; and topological approaches, including classification schemes of Tonnies and Durkheim. After brief analyses of these models, the author explicates his own theory of community, what he termed a "field theory." This, he explained, was based on four common characteristics taken from a work by Wilkinson [9]. For Wilkinson, a field was a holistic interaction nexus was unbounded, dynamic, and emergent. Preston argued that a "field" was different from a "social system" in several ways. First, the "concept of system" implied an inherent maintenance tendency, while the field concept made social and psychological concomitants to change its central focus. Second, boundary maintenance and the notion of a closed system were emphasized in the system model, whereas the field perspective emphasized community as an "emergent social field" [8, p. 56]. They key elements within the field were the actors, associations, and actions. The field could be analyzed at four levels: The ecological and demographic; cultural-institutional; social; and psychological or individual. Fields could be of various types, including pluralist-elitist (referring to their leadership structure); autonomous-coordinative (referring to their action styles); limited interest-multi-interest (referring to their coordinating associations); interventive-collaborative (referring to their relationship to the larger society).

According to Preston, each model was useful in directing policy for the CMHC. In this sense his work can be seen as being conciliatory and a new attempt at synthesis among models. According to him, the cultural level provided a basis for analysis of institutional structures in the community; the social level, for analysis or the relationship between program issues and local decision making; the psychological level, with issues of individual functioning. Planners using this model, it was suggested, should be able to deal with issues such as the power structure of the community, the impact of local initiatives or planned interventions, choice of leadership for CMHCs, relationships to classes in the community, and catchmenting.

Rather than assuming a unity among norms, values, and roles within the various associations existing in the community (association meaning interest groups much like those defined by Dahrendorf), Preston focused attention on the slippages and misalignments so obvious among such elements, a focus somewhat reminiscent of Merton's work on the slippages between cultural goals and structural means.

Although Preston went to some lengths to differentiate field theory from systems theory, in fact, the two seemed closely akin to one another. Both shared a claim to holism while actually breaking analysis into discrete, rather ahistorical subsystems. Both shared a claim to integrating actor and action, while actually reifying the actor and presenting him/her outside of ongoing interaction processes. (This latter corresponds rather closely to Parson's early work on the social act.) Preston never questioned the consensual basis of community, the legitimacy of authorities such as the policy or clergy representing themselves as agents of that consensus, or the assumption that society was self-maintaining, tending toward equilibrium.

In short, Preston had not replaced Parsons' social system, he had shifted the focus of attention from rigid structure to a more fluid accommodation among subsystems. Rather than starting with Parsons' jigsaw puzzle view of the social world into which each piece (personality, culture, society, the organism, for example) must be fit (see Chapter 2), Preston picked pieces at random and mused over their relationship to one another in a style reminiscent of Merton's middle-range functional analysis. Preston seemed to find that pieces of the social puzzle fit together poorly, sometimes leaving gaps, but he never doubted that all pieces eventually could be fit into this newly elastic puzzle-frame.

There was no questioning of class, mode of production, emergent liberated consciousness, conflict as the basis of history, or any other element of conflict analysis. There was no attempt at dialectical analysis, nor any at analysis of inherent contradictions—repulsion among pieces rather than attraction. Preston's analysis remained firmly in the consensual camp, despite the fact that the volume for which he wrote seemed to attempt to be presenting a broad overview of sociological theory in the CMHC literature.

The inclusion of Preston's essay in the volume might be seen as an example of a newly refined consensualism, if it were offset with a number of conflict sociological analyses. But, in fact, the conflict troops had disappeared over the hill by the mid 1970s. (See Chapter 4). Angry protests of the 1960s' conflict theorists were muted. Now the protests where phrased as reformist calls based on consensual community models.

Dunham

Another example of the 1970s articulation within the consensual camp, came in the works of Warren Dunham. Never one to mince words, Dunham had been producing warnings and criticisms about the direction of community psychiatry and community mental health for several decades. As early as 1965, he wrote a much quoted work

"Community Psychiatry: The Newest Therapeutic Bandwagon," [10] published in the *Archives of General Psychiatry*. In this essay Dunham attacked the expansion of psychiatry into the realm of social engineering and community development, areas he considered neither germane to psychiatry's role nor to psychiatric training.

In 1976, Dunham published *Social Realities and Community Psychiatry* [11]. In this collection of essays, including ones written earlier, Dunham explored the models and methods of community psychiatry. He explained that the CMHC movement had been heavily premised upon a systems model of society, which had been inappropriately used to expand traditional therapies into social engineering.

Not only was the model restrictive, but the view of community presented in community psychiatry education material was high idealized [1, p. 87].

> This image seems to consist, with its shifting perspective due to variations in income, of rows of neat little houses, each surrounded by a picket fence with geraniums on the window sills, with carefully tended lawns, well preserved and well cared for, stretching out away from the collection of stores which service the people in the community and with schools and churches scattered throughout the area. It is a community where people are friendly, where they support their local institutions, where they raise and care for their children, and where life goes on within a fixed rhythm year after year and generation after generation. In short, it is the kind of conception that Thornton Wilder portrays in *Our Town*. . . . These mythical communities, of course, have various problems but their citizens would always deal with them in an overtly, sensible, rational and humane fashion with varying degrees of success. Sometimes it seems to me that we have come to a point where many of us have become victims of our own propaganda.

Clearly, Dunham was upset over the impact of this "propaganda." His aim was to explore the model and its influence. But in doing so, he, like Preston, was unable to move beyond the consensual systems models which he attacked.

Dunham set out to investigate the sociological model underlying the field of community psychiatry. He posited two systems models: a rational systems model, in which parts could be individually manipulated to enhance the total structure; and the natural systems model, in which modification of any one part more clearly brought repercussions throughout the system [11, p. 127]. The first represents what I have discussed as the functional approach of Merton; the latter the systems approach of Parsons. (See Chapter 2). Both, however, fall into the consensual social systems of school of theory. Both systems models had far-reaching implications for the conceptualization of deviance. With any system forming the socio-ecological environment for an individual, changes in the system clearly influenced that individual. If the evolving system developed too much disequilibrium, this imbalance eventually created pathology in the individual. Dunham wrote that systems models were borrowed from the natural sciences and formed the basis of CMHC social engineering.

The systems model guided and limited the view of community by situating it within the conceptual framework of a consensually-based social system. (See Chapter 2.) It also limited and biased the conceptualization of deviance by judging normative conformity by a standard of hypothesized value consensus. (See Chapter 2.) The consensual basis of systems models also influenced policy recommendations. Rather than encouraging basic research on social reform, systems models tended to encourage elaborate listings of parts of the system, with little acknowledgement of the larger processes. This micro-analytical focus lent itself nicely to ahistorical, fragmentary views of social structure and social organization.

For example, Dunham himself set forth a list of sociological problems raised by the CMHC movement including the definition of limits and size of the population with analysis of its demography, analysis of bureaucracies involved with public support, issues of system centralization versus decentralization, problems of integrating new community centers with existing facilities, problems of the catchmenting concept and professional roles and authority, and finally, the issue of identifying the community itself [11, pp. 184-187]. As can be seen from this list, Dunham focused on exactly the kind of reformist administrative concerns addressed by Preston and by most consensual social planners. Rather than raising basic questions as to fundamental political economic power and control, as did conflict theorists, consensual theorists remained wedded to incremental reforms. Their concerns only skimmed along the surface of the existing societal order. Their rejection of prophetic sociology and acceptance of priestly reformism was reflected throughout their policy works, in defining community for measures of service, defining organizational systems of purposes of administration, and defining professional roles for the sake of the professionals themselves. The dark cloud of accountability floated over this analysis. Rather than addressing uncomfortable issues of capitalist profits and exploitation of labor, of emergent consciousness among non-conformers and contradictions in the mental health labor force itself, both Preston and Dunham preferred to address only issues of subsystem integration and re-equilibration of stability under the given political-economic order. The consensual basis of their theory permitted no other course. As long as they clung to the consensual model of society, including the role of legitimate authority and the evolutionary, basis of social change, they were trapped.

Their pseudo-critical consensual approach was adopted by quite a number of interest group theorists. Such theorists could sound like critics while suggesting only the mildest of reforms. They could remain priests while clothing themselves in prophetic garb. The pseudo-critical stance allowed for a suitably reformist tone to be adopted in analyses of the CMHC movement, yet it also facilitated comfortable working relations between applied scholars, administrators, politicians and others in the field. Questions, many questions, could be raised about the functioning of services and their accountability. Yet questions as to the interests served by the concept of accountability itself, about the capitalist marketplace and monopoly sector profits, were no longer raised in the elite literature. Consumers were no longer the angry black parents confronting Caplan a decade before. Consumers were artificial creations of applied scholars. They were mandated to be representative of "the community," and interest group theorists were only too happy to suggest how must artificial groups were to be defined, legitimated, and managed.

Nassi

The most clear cut debate between conflict and consensus in the community mental health literature during this period came in an exchange of articles on community control published in the *Journal of Community Psychology* in 1978. Alberta J. Nassi a member of the University of California at Davis Medical School faculty, set forth a conflict paradigm of community control, drawing on the work of Holton, New and Hessler in differentiating among: 1) *community involvement*, programs for the poor designed by professionals; 2) *community participation*, programs by the poor such as advisory boards; and 3) *true community control*, programs of the poor, implying not merely participation but control and power [12, p. 6]. Each of these corresponded to an ideological position, according to the author. The first corresponded to the traditional or conservative position; the second to the liberal reformist; and the third to the radical position. Nassi followed in the footsteps of former conflict authors whom she cited, such as Kunnes. (See Chapter 6.)

Nassi rejected the assumptions that society was based in value consensus and existing as a system in equilibrium. She adopted instead the conflict model of society defined through class conflict, with a division of labor reflecting control by the dominant class. The conflictual thrust to Nassi's argument was clearly echoed in her analysis of community control [12, p. 12]:

> The benefits of a shift of power to the local community would include: (a) a direct challenge to the prerogative of centralized bureaucracy to establish local policy; (b) a dramatic transformation and improvement in the health care service delivery system through accountability to the consumer and a transformation of tradition power relationships; (c) a mechanism for self-determination and the acquisition of greater competence, skills and resources; and (d) an alternative model of government and social decision making, which rejects the efficacy of representative but distant institutions to reflect popular aspirations in a given locale.

In (d), Nassi most directly suggested the heart of her concern, i.e. the need for an alternative political economic formation.

In the same issue of the Journal, in response to Nassi, several authors presented their own analyses of community control. Although labeling their approaches with a variety of names, a closer look revealed that each of these respondents was firmly entrenched in the consensual camp.

The first of these respondents, Donald Klein was the author of earlier works on field theory and the CMHC movement [13]. Klein agreed with Nassi that professional control of services had to be challenged, but warned that gaining community control would be a hard-fought contest. Despite his suspicion that professional control should be questioned, Klein revealed his consensual bias when he ended his discussion with: "In the meanwhile, one of the best means to enlist power on the side of the consumer is to help professionals gain a more enlightened grasp of their function and the function of the agencies in maintaining social inequities, including racism, in the larger society which supports them" [13, p. 18]. Klein's analysis did not carry beyond dissatisfaction with traditional professional autonomy to a more fundamental analysis of the political economic underpinnings of the current system. He seemingly believed that enlightened professionals could escape the hold of the infrastructure—their class, and that improved communication among consumers and professionals could overcome these differences.

Also responding to Nassi was Paul Dokecki a transactional analyst, who argued that social change would have to come slowly through all levels of the interactional processes [14]. Change would come through individual and professional transactions which produced outcomes either in harmony or opposed to values of the broader community and with a narrower community of family, peers, ethnic groups or the like. Dokecki argued that cultural slippages among these elements were the root cause of concern over change. He wrote [14, p. 20]:

> Application of the developmental theory to transactionally con-ceptualized mental health issues leads us to appreciate the developmental need for pursuing equilibration of assimilative (adjust the individual to society) and accommodative (help society change to incorporate new and potentially creative element) processes.

Dokecki rejected what he called "single-factor" approaches, and favored human development liaisons utilizing an ecological perspective to forge new transactional connections for human development. In this article he consistently invoked the consensual assumption that subsystems within the larger system needed to be reintegrated. The job of the interactional specialist, as he saw it, was to re-equilibrate these systems, not undermine them. Dokecki was very like the Mertonian con-sensual puzzle player who saw the need to stretch or shrink several of the puzzle pieces, but never attempted to rework the total design. (See Chapter 2.)

The third author in this debate adopted his analytical style from traditional consensual community sociology. In his "Community Con-trol in Gesellschaft World: A Comment," Karl Flaming suggested that Nassi's argument challenged the fundamental assumptions of indus-trialized society, especially their specialization and professionalization [15]. He argued that a gradual evolutionary process was needed "in which both the professional and the client are educated to understand each other regarding the processes and structure within which they find themselves" [15, p. 24]. Perhaps Nassi's avoidance of terms such as capitalism and socialism misled this author to think that she was discussing all industrialized societies, and that she was attacking specialization and professionalism across all systems. In fact, she was clearly invoking traditional conflictual criticism of specialization and professionalization under capitalism which served dominant interests in that particular political-economic system. Flaming's argument that a graduate evolutionary process was needed to correct the situation further underscored consensual thinking. Rather than criticizing the social structure in a fundamental sense, Flaming pointed toward improved communication as the key to community control, a view not unlike those expressed by both Klein and Dokecki. Flaming would have felt equally comfortable seated at the table of Mertonian puzzle enthusiasts, piecing together the consensual social system's puzzle.

This exchange of views was illuminating because it reflected the fading of conflict views in the 1970s. The cry of conflict voices in the late 1960s had been muffled, and when heard, it was immediately drowned out by a pseudo-plurality of essentially consensual voices. Whether employing the terminology of traditional sociological community analysis, field theory, or a social psychological interactional analysis, the consensual theme of the chorus was clear.[1]

Nassi, herself, responded to these critics by labeling them liberal reformers, reformers who acknowledged problems in the health care system but who were unwilling to challenge the political economic infrastructure which she saw causing them. In paraphrasing Bernstein et al. [16], she wrote [12, p. 27]:

> Liberal reformers argue that the problem of the mental health system can be remedied given enough time and the will to do so. They encourage community participation through exiting political channels. Informed administrators, better trained personnel, and an educated public portend the development of more responsive institutions. This analysis is basis on a short-sighted understanding of the realities of class, race, and power in the United States. Through these reforms the existing political and economic arrangements are secured, albeit in an ameliorated and regulated form, and capitalism is stoutly defended while working in the nave of enlightened reform.

To elaborate on the priest-prophet comparison, it can be said that the approach of applied consensualists in the 1970s was to take up the priestly worship of society while spicing their sermons with prophetic cries of injustice. By the mid-1970s, these consensual priests had

---

[1] It is interesting to note that this exchange took place in a journal of psychology rather than psychiatry. It may well have been that psychologists were more in tune with issues of the social, having escaped the medical model.

established their own denominational cliques by articulating specialized terminology of various consensual subschools such as transactional analysis and also by politically allying themselves with varieties of
consensual special interest models.

INTEREST GROUP THEORY: CONSUMERS

Chu and Trotter

The use of consensual interest group theory by the middle-class
consumer movement was widespread in this decade. The foremost
advocate of this approach, Ralph Nader, turned his attention toward
the CMHC movement early in the 1970s. In 1974, *The Madness Establishment* was published by Chu and Trotter under the sponsorship of
the Nader organization [4].

Chu and Trotter presented their analysis in the manner of inves-
tigative reporters, creating an image of truth seekers hot on the trail of
the real CMHC movement. One of their first targets was catchmenting
which they felt allowed centers to deny services to persons outside of a
particular geographic zone. Another major criticism was the ineffective
operation of citizen boards. Such groups, Chu and Trotter felt, were
given only the most minimal advisory role in policy.

Despite criticizing catchmenting and ineffective citizen boards, the
authors were not able to build a unified critique of why the CMHC
movement failed to live up to expectations. Chu and Trotter clung to a
view that consumer interests represented community interests.
The best they could say was that consumers, for example, the needy
or minorities, should be actively sought out and included in CMHC
planning and administrative responsibilities.

The author's lack of understanding of, or at least of the application
of, alternative social theory led them to assign blame for the
movement's failure to elitist politicians and bureaucrats. They investigated what they saw as the CMHC movement weaknesses by
documenting problems in the implementation of regulations and in
bureaucratic procedures. Chu and Trotter failed to provide a systematic analysis of why such regulations and such procedures were
developed in the first place, whom they served, and why they consistently fell short of change.

In their final chapter, aptly entitled, "Innovation Without Change,"
the authors reviewed the major points of their analysis [4, pp. 202-203]:

In retrospect the community mental health centers program was vastly oversold, the original goals quickly perverted—possibly because of the contradictory assumption that revolutionary change could be successfully wrought by those professionals and politicians with a vested interest in maintaining the status quo. At any rate, CMHC feebly communicated the original intent of the program to state and local officials; failed to coordinate the location of the centers with other HEW health and social-welfare efforts; made little attempt to train (or retain) people for community work; avoided funding centers outside the narrow interests of the medical profession; did not engage consumers in the planning or operation of centers; and made only the most perfunctory evaluation of the program's performance. As a result, community mental health centers tend to involve only a renaming of conventional psychiatry, a collection of traditional clinical services that are in most cases not responsive to the needs of large segments of the community, and which often leave community people indifferent, sometimes antagonistic.

The model here was of professional crusaders allied with consumers, both locked in a battle with the bureaucrats and the professional elite who were seen as controlling CMHC services. What was missing was an analysis of these providers and consumers within the larger context of political and economic arena. Chu and Trotter's assumption seemed to be that, if only the proper consumers, the poor and minorities, for example, could have their say in legislation, regulations, and implementation, then innovative services would be developed. This was typical of the liberal view of reform and was the basis of much of the planning legislation implemented by the federal government in the 1970s, for example, the Health Systems Agency (HSA) legislation, P.L. 93-641. This liberal reformist stance was supported by the consensual systems model of society. It was assumed that interest groups disagreed because of differing vested interests, but there was no consistent exploration of class-based interests, interests which historically rose and fell under varying political economic pressures. There was only a keen awareness of the need for accessible, humanized services spread to needy populations. There was also no systematic questioning of differing ideologies of health and illness related to historically fixed classes or of the role of "legitimate authorities" in supporting the prevailing modes of thought. Rather, there was only discontent with the lack of pluralism in decision making, a pluralism assumed to be supplied by adding equal numbers of providers and consumers to

CMHC boards of directors. The message was: Give consumers information, knowledge about what's happening, and they will take responsibility. Give them a chance to sit on legislative panels or advisory groups and they will produced innovative solutions to these problems. The possibility that elite spheres of interest controlled knowledge production within mental health, or that class differences systematically excluded persons from control was not addressed. In many ways, Chu and Trotter's work bore a striking resemblance to the earlier work of Caplan. (See Chapter 5.) These two seemingly divergent schools of thought, i.e. psychiatric consultation versus consumerism shared a heritage of applied consensual social theory. The solution offered by each to inequality of services and non-responsiveness to change was to bring all elements into an open dialogue about decision making. Through such dialogue, and through improved administration, management and accountability, services would be humanized. Unlike the conflict argument which systematically linked control of services to the interests of class-based elites, consensual reformists saw interests as potentially equal participants in social system functioning.

INTEREST GROUP THEORY: PROVIDER

Bolman

It is important to note that the two groups defined as oppositional by the reformist literature, "consumers" and "providers," both adopted applied consensual thought. While Chu and Trotter took up the cause of the consumer, others were more interested in reaching the provider.

In the same year that Chu and Trotter published *The Madness Establishment*, 1974, Leopold Bellak, a prominent figure in the CMHC movement, was bringing out a new version of his landmark work, *Handbook of Community Psychiatry and Community Mental Health*, originally published in 1964. The new version, *A Concise Handbook of Community Psychiatry and Community Mental Heath* revealed that Bellak had retreated from his earlier pronouncement that community psychiatry represented a revolution in psychiatry [17]. Now the author wrote that the CMHC movement had advanced beyond the first ten "heroic" years of the movement and was in a phase of stocktaking. What the movement represented was a variety of treatments focused on a variety of treatment groupings. The new book reflected a belief in the correctness of interest group pluralism as a way to understand consumer needs. Consumers included the elderly, children, and drug abusers—groups targeted for treatment in CMHC regulations.

The interest group emphasis is nowhere more clearly voiced than in the last essay in Bellak's volume *"Policy Aspects of Consumer Participation,"* by William M. Bolman [18]. Bolman's purpose in his essay seemed to be to discuss issues of power and control for professionals in the movement. He reviewed varieties of what he called "health-illness ideologies" and discussed conflicts of priorities in service delivery. In a typical grab bag approach, he included in his review of CMHCs a brief discussion of problems intrinsic and extrinsic to centers. Intrinsic issues included the choice of community representative for boards, board members' roles, new types of community activities, and possible rearrangement of professional priorities. Extrinsic issues included definitional issues of health and illness and the definitions of professional roles.

In the midst of this wide ranging discussion, complete with several short case studies, the author mentioned numerous interest groups, such as blacks, poor, and professionals. With no explicit theory to guide his analysis, Bolman offered typologies of people with interests in CMHCs, ideologies, and types of involvement.

The first typology was actually a partial list of pertinent interest groups. (See Table 5.) In his typology of interests, Bolman included a wide range of persons interested in community mental health. Each type of person was defined through his/her connection with the issue of mental illness. The author suggested that professionals manifested a wide range of interests themselves, and, in certain cases joined with other community care givers in serving their community. In addition, helpful citizens, citizens with specialized interests, or what he termed obstructive citizens, at one time or another joined with professionals to follow common interests. What the author failed to achieve was a systematic representation of historically defined groups, groups which significantly differed form one another on criteria beyond their acquaintance with mental illness. Failing this type of analysis, Bolman was confined to his rather *ad hoc* description typology of interests.

This shortcoming was more clearly reflected in his topology of types of involvement. (See Table 6.) Here the reader learned that interest groups could also be classified by the reaction of professionals to clients. Professionals might choose to manipulate, therapeutize, give over control, etc., to various client groups. This typology too remained at the level of description rather than analysis and was reminiscent of

Table 5. A Typology of People with an Interest in
Community Mental Health Programs

Person	Interests
The mental health professional	A wide variety of interests and motives ranging from self-interest to technical and humanistic concerns, variously dedicated to earning a living, being helpful, treating patients, consulting, preventive efforts, etc.
Other professionals and community care givers who encounter mental health problems in their work	Assistance in making their own work easier, whether by gaining more competence (as via consultation) or by referral for treatment of needy clients.
Citizens with a sense of civic obligation and a general interest in mental health	Generalized interest in being helpful, tending to be deferential to mental health professionals, especially physicians.
Citizens who have encountered mental health problems, e.g., with friends, relatives, children or selves	Specialized interest, often critical of mental health system.
Citizens who mistrust the goals or activities of mental health, generally of an ultraconservative orientation	Mostly concerned with obstructing, criticizing, and exposing so as to block mental health programs.
Members of minority groups concerned with powerlessness, inequality, and unresponsive social institutions.	Initially concerned with acquiring control and self-determination, then concerned with changing programs to meet minority needs.

Source: William M. Bolman [18, p. 223].

Table 6. Types of Involvement

Level	Type	Meaning
1	Manipulation	Professionals consult with citizens to gain political support and allies. No other changes are intended.
2	Therapy	Professionals, usually via someone delegated for the job, consult with client-citizens to help them become "less alienated."
3	Informing	Professionals meet with cooperative citizen representatives to inform them of plans, problems, and needs in order to maintain support.
4	Consultation	Professionals meet with a variety of citizen representatives to ask their advice about plans, problems, and needs.
5	Placation	Professionals meet with militant citizen representatives to prevent them from obstructing plans.
6	Partnership	Professionals and all kinds of citizens participate equally in making plans, solving problems, and meeting needs.
7	Delegated power	Professionals relinquish control of one or more specific programs to a community group.
	Citizen control	Professionals work as employees under the direction of a citizen board.

Source: William M. Bolman [18, p. 228].

Panzetta's discussion of community based on a market model of supply and demand.

But Bolman went beyond Panzetta. Rather than advising professionals that their services were subject to laws of supply and demand, as Panzetta did, Bolman acknowledged that professionals could take a more active role themselves. Now, with the experience of the 1960s behind them, professionals were advised that they could react to interests, managing them with a variety of social control techniques. The professional could now take the offensive, become the active focus of legitimation for the interests.

To what end did Bolman describe types of citizen involvement? One reason might have been to chide professionals into recognition of their positions of power and control. In reviewing the outcome of citizen participation in policy, Bolman concluded [18, p. 228],

> Indeed, it is embarrassing and/or exasperating to observe the degree of both conscious and unconscious condescension exhibited by well-meaning professionals in trying to deal with the new citizen groups.

While recognizing that many health services were distributed and controlled on the basis of class and ethnic differences, Bolman never incorporated these class and ethnic differences into his own topologies. The liberal reformist tone of this interest group theorist could be acceptable to fellow practitioners as long as it was couched in consensual terminology. Were Bolman to adopt the rhetoric of conflict sociology, capitalism-socialism, dominant class-working class, exploitation-liberation, for example, it is doubtful whether many professionals would have been willing to listen. The annoyance at arrogance, an annoyance conveyed by Chu and Trotter and by Bolman was enough to satisfy both a disgruntled middle class and federal bureaucrats who were determined to reprivitize the mental health service market. Yet these critiques deflected attention away from the underlying political and economic dynamics of the mental illness market.

Regester

Another variation on the theme of consensual interest groups was presented at about the same time as Chu and Trotter and Bolman were presenting their works. David C. Regester published his work in the *American Journal of Public Health* [19]. In his article, "Community Mental Health—For Whose Community?," Dr. Regester presented eight conceptual models of community and their implications for such issues as staff awareness of needs, effect on programming, and the role of citizens. (See Table 7.)

In taking a close look at these categories, it could be seen the they summarize most of the models adopted within the movement's literature over the preceding decade. Absent again however, was any conflict model. Number 1, the geographical area, was the catchment model.

Table 7. Determining Criteria for the Target Population

Conceptual Model of Community	Criteria Determining Target Population
1. Geographical area	Based on residence within geographical limits. Creates problem regarding appropriateness of service to transients (alcoholics, migrant workers, etc.). Those closer to one CMHC may be excluded from service because they live outside the catchment area, thus causing undue inconveniences of travel, time, etc. Boundaries which result may be appropriate geographically, but questionable by other standards, which could "well be a source for precipitating emotional illness rather than preventing it."
2. Majority	The greatest number of people. Greater emphasis on numbers of people than on kinds of problems served or quality of service.
3. Vocal minority	Those who are sufficiently vocal and potentially powerful politically. Staff may be used to advance sometimes conflicting objectives of certain politically influential or needy groups. Importance of consultation and education function as a feedback mechanism between the community and the CMHC to ensure quality, breadth, and appropriateness of services.
4. Society-at-large	Determined by problems common to all. Focus of concern on problems, rather than geographical or numerical considerations, is considered desirable from a mental health viewpoint.
5. Common body	Determined by specific, commonly shared population attributes. Leads to ingrouping and outgrouping, cliques, rejection of others because of differences, usually not productive mental health consequences.

Table 7. (Cont'd.)

Conceptual Model of Community	Criteria Determining Target Population
6. Feeling of belongingness	Those who share feelings of acceptance of others, regardless of personal attributes. Significant mental health goal (acceptance of others) incorporated in target definition.
7. Elitist	Determined primarily by staff attitudes. Deficient in mental health concepts. Limitations on clientele may conflict with community concerns. Implication of possible staff indifference to community concerns.
8. System of mutual interactions	Only those mutually involved in relationships. Sound mental health goal (facilitation of relationships between systems and people) incorporated in target definition. May result in service only to interacting systems, thus isolating others (sometimes easier to work with mutually involved systems than to initiate interactions where none have existed).

Source: David Regester [19, p. 889].

The second model, termed "majority," was much like Panzetta's market model insofar as numbers of consumers or clients were the focus of concern. The third, "vocal minority," hinted as struggles from the 1960s and addressed the role of consultation in linking the clients to CMHC policy. The "common body" category reflected a return to the old consensual systems ideal. The "feeling of belongingness" derived from Howe's community of consciousness. The "elitist" model mirrored contemporary language concerning struggles between consumer interests and provider interests. The "system of mutual interactions" drew on both general systems models and the ecological models. Although Regester gathered together a great many of the previous approaches to community, he did not get to the underlying social theory informing them. He did not realize that all were variations on the consensual theme.

Table 8. Effect of Conceptual Models of Community
on Target Population

Conceptual Model of Community	Effect on Target Population
1. Geographical area	Concern with territoriality, whether explicit or implicit, tends to alienate clients who are naturally more concerned with their problems, and who find such restrictions arbitrary and detrimental to the public concern. Leininger reinforces this view: ". . . some punitive artificial boundaries . . . could well be a major source for precipitating emotional illness rather than preventing it. . . ."
2. Majority	Appropriate emphasis on the majority of population leads to concern with assessing the effect on the majority. To the extent qualitative evaluation is overlooked, this model can lead to the use of misleading evaluative criteria, such as the "numbers game" which is so often played. The illogic of this game is that program success is directly related to the number of clients processed. A more positive aspect of this game is that it can justify programs to politicians who can make or break programs because of reliance on public monies.
3. Vocal minority	Results in discriminatory and possibly also prejudicial service. In such models, there is always a "winner" and a "loser" in the sense that some factions are attended to while others are not. If there is a failure to discriminate effectively, then resulting prejudicial service will be detrimental to the mental health of the total target population.
4. Society-at-large	Enhances mental health concepts, thus leading to a broad based philosophical approach which should affect community at many different levels— limited only by the diversity of professionals included in such a CMHC.

Table 8. (Cont'd.)

Conceptual Model of Community	Effect on Target Population
5. Common body	Such a conceptual restriction is likely to lead to infighting among community factions, stereotypic thinking about others, inflexibility of attitudes toward mental health, and a decreasing tolerance for individual differences, obviously deleterious to community mental health. However, maintenance of stability and deviance control could be considered a desirable effect within this model.
6. Feeling of belongingness	Promotes valid mental health ideals (capacity to adapt to change, tolerance for deviance, etc.). The focus on feelings and attitudes is felt to be desirable goal, which if implemented would be quite beneficial to the target population.
7. Elitist	Delimits clientele by some selective process, usually very subtle. Effect of intellectually superior and authoritarian air of staff is highly suspect in these days of grassroots applications favoring paraprofessionals, indigenous workers, peer counselors, etc. Felzer cites examples of programs of a socially active CMHC whose interests do correspond with those of the community: "Organization of a tenant strike, protests to city council about police and busing problems in (a) city," etc.
8. System of mutual interactions	Model appropriately expands conceptualization from intrapsychic to sociological, ecological, and public health realms, thus potentially increasing breadth of impact on target population. Pursley et al. illustrate how a systems approach can be effectively applied, giving examples especially relevant to school systems.

Source: David Regester [19, p. 892].

Regester did perform a useful service by systematically listing implications of his models, for 1) staff characteristics (for example, the vocal minority focused staff attention on specialty areas); 2) awareness of community needs (for example, the vocal minority created linkages in these groups and also caused the staff to distribute services like a "political football"); and 3) the effect on the target population (for example, the vocal minority could result in discriminatory and possibly prejudicial services by winning services form non-vocal interests).

The consensual orientation of the author came through loud and clear in the last stage of his analysis, the effect of the models on the target population. (See Table 8.)

The author suggested that the catchment model might tend to alienate clients, the majority might lead to the misuse of evaluation criteria, the vocal minority model might result in discrimination, the common body model might be restrictive and lead to infighting.

None of these models fundamentally challenged the right of mental health professionals to define deviance. Regester's language of interest groups lent an aura of critical insight by focusing attention on varieties of CMHC services. Still this analysis lacked bite; it lacked heuristic importance because of its overlapping and rather arbitrary listing of interests.

While failing to add much new insight, these typologies did fulfill a function. By their existence, they suggested that CMHC authors, producers of knowledge for the movement, were continuing to grapple with the slippery concept of community. These lists made it seem that professionals in the centers were getting closer to finding true community representatives to guide them in their task of serving the whole community. This literature also could be drawn upon as safe training material with which to sensitize staff to the pluralistic conceptualization of community thereby answering criticisms from consumer advocates. These typologies of interests lent an air of responsible applied scholarship to the mid-1970s' literature while obscuring the absence of earlier conflict-based criticism. Rather than answering conflict critics directly, and thereby legitimating their questions, mainstream CMHC authors adopted a shallow critical tone of their own devising through listings of special interests. They defined a myriad of interests and called these "the community." They presented the reader with what seemed to be a plurality of models, but what was actually a narrowly drawn, pseudo-plurality of interest groups growing out of a middle range consensual approach.

CONSULTATION AND SPECIAL INTERESTS

The policy implications of interest group theorizing were clearly mirrored in the literature on consultation, a literature based in pragmatic applications of CMHC theory. Earlier consultation attempts had focused on bringing the good news of mental health and social control to non-mental health authorities such as school administrators and the police. In the late 1960s, CMHC consultants had been forced to go beyond cooperative consultations in which they dealt with their professional counterparts, and to mediate confrontatins between professionals and their angry clients. By the 1970s, the consultation literature, too, began to fill with lists and typologies. The intent seemed to be to legitimate certain "community" interests and to exclude others. In this literature lists served to add the semblance of detail and precision to the concept of community. When CMHC authors went out to act in "the community" armed with these lists, they could feel content that they knew whom they were facing.

In 1975, Mannimo et al. published an account of an NIHC sponsored Mental Health Study Center in Prince George's County, Maryland [20]. Consultation through this center included work with the police, schools, courts, hospitals and other health agencies, industry, and the military. Any consensual framework would identify these as legitimate community interests. Likewise, Plog and Ahmed in 1977 suggested to consultants that they work with schools, welfare agencies, criminal justice agencies, churches, and the like [21].

ECOLOGY AND MULTIPLE MODELS

The community psychology literature remained vigorous in its explorations in theory beyond the late 1970s and into the 1980s. But it, too, was full of elaborations on earlier models. [22]. Heller and Monahan followed in this growing literature with their *Psychology and Community Change* in which they explored the idea of environmental feedback within the ecological community model [23]. They suggested that community change could take three major forms: 1) consultation which assumed a "within" the system strategy and would help existing agencies to work more effectively; 2) developing alternatives to existing community agencies, and intervention which would be especially appropriate when many identified needs were going unmet; and 3) organizing community-based groups of activists to redistribute power in the community. The authors felt that the choice of strategy depended on such variables as the homogeneity of the community, the extent of strain, and whether the strain was in the majority or the minority population. They also presented a rather detailed discussion of differences between community development based on such tactics as education versus the tactics of social action. The latter was identified as more overtly wed to conflict. Despite the talk of organizing activists, the concluding chapter brought the reader back to the ideal of ultimately reducing community strain through enhancing citizen participation and social cohesion.

These authors strayed further than most from the priestly model in emphasizing historically-based inherent struggles over the redistribution of power and control. They also envisioned an activist role in social change for social scientists who would use empirical evidence to give voice to unheard concerns. Interestingly enough, the authors noted that some psychologist wished to disassociate themselves from the term "community mental health" because it had become too closely linked to psychiatry. Community psychology, it was argued, included concerns beyond traditional psychiatry boundaries. It was plainly stated that psychologists wanted to avoid inappropriate medical overtones [23, p. 21].

A year later, in 1978, Mann published his *Community Psychology: Concepts and Applications* [24]. This was one of the fullest analyses of the diverse models which had, by the end of the decade, come to be represented in the community mental health literature. Although the prophetic conflict model was not mentioned, Mann provided a much fuller explication of the conceptual links between multiple priestly models, their implicit assumptions about community, and the intervention strategies their authors proposed. As Mann stated [24, p. xi],

> The history of community psychology shows a change from an initial concern with the application of psychology in the community to a broadened conception of a psychology about the community in a relatively brief period of time.

The first of Mann's models was mental health which included crisis intervention and consultation in the Caplan mode. The usual site of these interventions was the community mental health center. Within this model, community was conceptualized in terms of personal or interpersonal relationships within a geographic area. As the author correctly noted, this model assumed global values and rational decision making, along with an inherent social stability in the community. It was a restatement of the catchment idea.

The second model, termed the organizational model, was patterned on the work of Kurt Lewin and others in sensitivity training. Intervention based on this model was usually focused on organizational consultation. Community, within this model was seen as a set of organizations. Value was placed on face to face interaction, power sharing, and change arising from a special group atmosphere reflecting the freeing of interpersonal expectations and behaviors. It was akin to the transactional or field model.

Mann's third model was social action. This was associated with the social movements of the earlier decades and focused on organizing indigenous groups, often non-professionals, to share power more equitable with the given power structure. The community model assumed here, according to Mann, was defined by a particular constituency and not a social system. Change occurred through mobilization for power. This came closest to the earlier humanist conflict ideal.

Mann's last model was termed the ecological model. Here a central concept was "life space." Assumptions included the idea that community was an ecosystem based on interdependence, the cycling of resources, adaptation, and succession. Intervention strategies depended on the varying conditions of the ecosystem.

Perhaps the most intriguing aspect of Mann's work was the documentation of the multiplicity of models growing out of the generally socially conscious profession of psychology as opposed to a more reductionistic psychiatry. Another interesting aspect of the work was its lack of overt emphasis on the historical contexts of varying approaches. The reader was left to wonder what gave rise to one or another of the models, and why one was fashionable at a certain time rather than another. The underlying assumptions were never traced to their political economic roots.

EVALUATION RESEARCH AS LEGITIMATION OF SPECIAL INTERESTS

Although evaluation research as a tool of the social sciences had a lengthy history, the application of evaluation to the CMHC movement hadn't begin in earnest until the 1970s. The accountability frenzy had by this time been institutionalized into research offices in every CMHC.

In typical CMHC evaluation research, "community" was broken down into traditional clusters of variables reflecting such sociodemographic characteristics as marital status, sex, income, age, ethnicity, etc. These social indicators were meant both as markers for assumed need and as tools for measuring community access to care. Patient profiles were compared with demographic profiles of the catchment area in an attempt to find under served areas or interests.

NIMH in the mid-1970s began strongly advocating the use of census tract data in evaluations by all centers. In the spring of 1974, the federal Alcohol, Drug Abuse and Mental Health Administration sponsored a conference which was later published under the title, *Program Evaluation Alcohol, Drug Abuse, and Mental Health Services* [25]. Papers from the conference included several variations on the theme of evaluating community. One of the most comprehensive approaches was by Morrison and Sundel [26], "Development of a Community Assessment Strategy for Program Evaluation in a Comprehensive Human Service Delivery System." In this article the authors spelled out the uses to which administrators put data, including determining needs and usage, length of stay, numbers of new clients per month, etc.; uses of the data for prevention, for outreach, consultation, community education; for treatment such as staff education. The data collected on the community included population characteristics such as ethnicity, age and sex; family/non-family characteristics such as household size, *"normal* family life index" (my italics refer to percentage of husband/ wife households and children under 18 living with parents), matriarch index, marital status, family life cycle (number dependents in home), persons not in families; social characteristics, such as education, employment, occupational status; economic characteristics, such as employment, family income, families below poverty, persons below poverty housing characteristics, such as value of housing, year-round occupation, mobility, and condition of housing [26, pp. 165-167]. In addition to this information, the survey also made use of NIMH suggested comparisons with census tract data.

This and similar studies of "the community" [27, 28] divided the catchmented area into defined units to which services could be directed, for which needs could be assessed, and to which the center could say it was accountable.

A similar but more detailed use of census-tract analysis was discussed by Bloom in his 1975 work, *Changing Patterns of Psychiatric Care* [29]. Here the emphasis was on subarea analysis using traditional demographic data, such as age, sex, Spanish surname; family characteristics, such as number of young children, people living alone, married women in the labor force; housing characteristics, such

as owner-occupied units and single units; socio-economic characteristic, including income and unemployment; personal disruption
measured by delinquency, suicide, school dropouts, and marital disruption. In addition, Bloom added a measure of community participation,
including library card holders, YMCA membership, golf club membership, and public health nursing visits [5].

Through such operationalizations, community was concertized and
reified—it was made measurable and available for scientific research.
At the same time the unsettling questions of linking research to one's
theoretical assumptions could be obscured. Totally absent was any
attempt to develop research methods which derived from conflict
theory, looking at class as relations to the means of production rather
than the consensual socio-economic status (SES) indicators. History as
approached in such evaluation efforts was not the history of class
struggles, emergent conflicts were not the basis for community interaction, and class analysis from a conflict view could be ignored. By
defining variables ahistorically using cross-sectional survey methods,
the historical class struggles which troubled authors in the late 1960s
were replaced with the rhetoric of statistical technique. No longer were
there questions as to how to deal with an angry black neighborhood,
but how to properly enumerate black heads of household. Rather than
musing over the process of schooling as social control and its relationship to the politics and economy of the times, authors simply looked at
schooling as a source of variables for measures of noncompliance or
community pathology—numbers of days missed from school or number
of school dropouts. Rather than addressing questions relating to the
emergent role of women in the market and in the home, evaluation
researchers measured female heads of households or numbers of working mothers and assumed these reflected something about family disruption.

In 1974, an Evaluation and Program Implementation Division was
established in the Office of Management and Budget (OMB) in
Washington. In 1975, CMHCs were mandated by new federal amendments to include in their budgets support for evaluation research at a
level equal to 2 percent of the preceding year's budget. Evaluation
research had arrived.

At the same time, accessibility, availability, continuity of care,
cost control—all replaced the earlier concern with community participation in planning. The new focus of concern was on documenting these characteristics of services in the community-census tract-
catchment area.

Volumes on how to meet the demands of the OMB and the new regulations proliferated. A typical example was *Trends in Mental Health Evaluation* [30] from a conference held in 1975. In a refreshingly frank approach, these authors included a chapter entitled, "What Congress Really Wants: A Guide to Evaluating Program Effectiveness with Example from a Canadian Context" [30, pp. 61-71]. The political overtones of this research were always clear, and everyone was looking to Washington to lead the way.

In 1977, the publication of *Evaluating Community Mental Health Services: Principles and Practice* provided a look at what the Staff College of NIMH was teaching its own employees about evaluation [31]. Major topics included: management information systems, assessing needs, evaluation strategies, cost-effectiveness analysis, and evaluation leading to organization change. In this work it was noted that, by law, the centers had to turn out annual program evaluation reports. These were to include measurable specific objectives. The intent was clear, to provide neat management targets and objective criteria for meeting them.

Program characteristics which were to be reported included: cost of episode of indirect and direct care; number and rates of catchment area residents' use of service element; client age, sex, family income, race, and geographic subarea; availability of services, defined as services available to population, awareness of services, defined as knowledge by the local population and community caretakers about the services; acceptability, defined as use; accessibility, defined as ease of reaching the center with reference to time, geography, finances, psychological and sociocultural issues, impact of indirect services of consultation and education on program goals; effectiveness of reducing inappropriate institutionalization; and impact on the mental health and related problems of the residents of the catchment area [31, pp. 449-451]. An impressive list indeed! But with so much detail the whole was obscured. How could an uninitiated critic now begin to challenge the scientific or the theoretical basis of "community?"

Another interesting evaluation undertaken in the early 1970s, and published in 1981 was authored by Dorwart and Meyers [32], who found encouragement in the work and person of Gerald Caplan. As one would expect from a work in the Caplan tradition, this investigation adopted a model of community which conceptualized community as a consensual social system, one involving communication, social control, socialization, cohesion and differentiation [32, p. 22]. The authors specified that their evaluation data, following on a community model which characterized community as an entity unto itself rather than as a collection of individuals. Dorwart and Meyers consciously adopted what they termed a social-ecological perspective which "implies that demographic and social system characteristics of local areas are related to the activity of social agencies in an area" [32, p. 78]. This approach to community, thoroughly priestly in tone and content, echoed the Parsonian social system approach.

Dorwart and Meyers focused their evaluation on understanding how community characteristics helped explain the accomplishment, thoughts, and actions of community mental health advisory boards in Massachusetts. They interviewed board presidents, sent questionnaires to board members, and carried out several in-depth case studies. Their dependent variables included inter-organizational cooperation, attitudes of board members toward the boards, and general accomplishments. This last category included service creation and improvement, outside resource mobilization, local autonomy, and coordination of services [32, p. 86].

Their strongest statistical association came in the correlation between areas high in social disorganization and the dependent variable of service creation. Social disorganization was operationalized as including measures of social pathology, family instability, and social welfare recipiency [32, p. 86]. As the authors themselves point out, it was not surprising to find that citizens in such areas would place a high priority on providing new and better services. From a social control standpoint, it might be hypothesized that such areas posed the highest potential for disruption and so required services as vehicles for control. Interestingly enough, one conclusion of the study was that citizen boards aided in bypassing the politization of appointment of CMHC directors. This did not mean that citizen boards represented interests different from the professional service deliverers—a topic of debate since the inception of such boards. In fact, consistent with the consensual tradition which they represented, Dorwart and Meyers concluded that citizen boards needed to foster close cooperation between themselves, the CMHC board and staff, and to enter into coalitions with the professionals [32, pp. 135-137]. By the end of the decade, the alliance between applied social science evaluators and the leaders of the CMHC movement was thriving [33-35].

Despite the increasing complexity and sophistication of evaluation methodological, no less a notable than Daniel X. Freedman, a well-known psychiatrist, wrote in 1970 that [36, p. 179]:

> Trivial assertions and self-serving haphazard countings are called evaluation . . . and prevail over a handful of top flight and serious investigations in the assessment area.

In 1976, the movement by special interests and others to consolidate the mental health service market on the federal level found a receptive audience in the person of the new President's wife, Rosalyn Carter. She was appointed honorary chair of a national commission to study mental health needs and draft new mental health legislation.

THE PRESIDENT'S COMMISSION ON MENTAL HEALTH

President Carter established this commission in 1977 with the charge to review the metal health needs of the nation and make recommendations on meeting those needs. Task Panels were set up on a variety of topic areas including community supports, the service system, insurance, personnel, basic rights, prevention and the knowledge base. From each Task Panel, recommendations were culled and compiled in a *Report to the President* [37], which was accompanied by three volumes of Task Panel reports. The entire four volume work was published in 1978.

Early on, the commission members realized they were laying the foundation for new legislation which would replace the CMHC acts. The task of translating the Report into congressional action took several years, coming to fruition in the 1981 passage of the short-lived Mental Health Systems Act.

Taken as a reflection of the sociological sophistication of federal policy makers, the *President's Commission Report* revealed a small degree of improvement over the knowledge base of the participants in the development of the original CMHC Act. Rather than adopting a rather shallow model of community such as the doctor's marketplace (See Chapter 5), the authors of this new work carved up that marketplace into public and private zones overlaid with a myriad of special interests—what might have been expected due to the developments in the literature in the 1970s. Those elements of the existing sociocultural order with the strongest ties to the mental health service system, such as the police, schools, and religious groups, were designated as part of the "natural order" of society. In the second volume, The Report called for a major new federal initiative in community mental health to [37, p. 144]:

Recognize and strengthen the natural networks to which people belong and on which they depend—families, kin, kith, friendship, and neighborhood social networks; work relationships; religious denominations and congregations; and self-help groups and other voluntary associations based on principles of intimacy and mutual aid. Identify and strengthen the potential social support functions of formal care giving institutions.

Improve the linkages between natural helping networks and the more formal sources of help—professional and institutional.

Develop educational strategies to inform the general public and care giving professionals on the nature and function of natural helping networks and on the importance of attachments and mutuality for well-being.

Initiate research to provide national data periodically on social support and on natural helping networks in American society, to monitor the direction and magnitude of changes in these aspects of American life, and to increase knowledge of how best to attain the above objectives.

Here, as in the remainder of the Report, the emphasis was on maintaining the stability of the existing social order. Cooperation rather than conflict was assumed to be the natural basis for human interaction, and "natural" patterns of human solidarity depended on warmth, love, and understanding. Families, friends, religions, the law and mutual aid groups were portrayed as natural outgrowths of this warmth, and extensions of the consensual value basis of society.

No where was there recognition of conflict growing out of basic political economic inequalities, of divisions among the population which represented class-based exploitation or of competing ideologies. Instead, the assumption was clearly one of sociocultural consensus reflecting the natural order of community, stabilized and strengthened through mental health services.

One diagram in the Report showed a mutually supportive relationship among Professional Helping Networks (including schools, religious institutions, social service agencies, hospitals, CMHCs, among others), and Natural Helping Networks, (including the family, clergy, teachers, self-help groups, unions, and voluntary associations, among others) [37, p. 161]. This rather arbitrary listing of collectivities and formal authorities seemed to suggest more about the interests represented in the mental health service market, and their standing in the consciousnesses of the Report's authors, than it did about social structure or change.

Much of the work of the Task Panels involved dealing with sociological models. Unfortunately, there was no critical analysis of these models or their assumptions. A section on religion focused on maximizing the influence of clergy as mental health workers. Another section focused on extending the role of schools in working with troubled youth. For example, one program, mentioned as a model, had been founded by judges, educators, and others, "to address the problems of youth alienation, and to promote opportunities for youth to assume responsibility and socially useful roles in their local schools and community" [37, p. 199]. No discussion was presented on whether such alienation could be a legitimate expression of exploitation, or of the role of the schools and courts in social control. This avoidance of social control issues was also seen in other sections of the Community Support Task Panel Report dealing with using the justice system to strengthen families and communities.

Nowhere in the work was there recognition of the special qualities related to building consciousness. Gray Panthers were lumped together with government sponsored Indian aid groups, and both were seen as extensions of the mental health service system. Apparently, the conflict voices of the 1960s had made no lasting impression on the authors of this document. It stood as a federal reaffirmation of the soundness of the existing mental health market. *The President's Commission Report* signalled the power of consensual special interest models in serving the needs of the market and State at the end of the decade. Rather than continually having to justify new positions for funding, representatives of special interest groups could now identify themselves as spokespersons for "natural" elements of the social structure, as extenders of professional services, and as colleagues of legitimate authorities who supported the evolutionary growth of American society.

Perhaps Daniel X. Freedman's essay, "Community Mental Health: Slogan or New Direction," [38] provided the best summarization of the movement at the end of the decade. Dr. Freedman saw that despite the "metaphorical morass" encountered by those exploring the meaning of community mental health, the movement did produce facilities and services founded through public health-minded officials at NIMH [38, p. 179].

According to that author, the movement followed rather naturally from the earlier practitioners of moral treatment. But the federal planning motivation evolved to the point of using the CMHC movement to develop a type of "socialized psychiatric care—fare in advance of such arrangements for general health care" [38, p. 184].

In addition to the political problems within this effort, it raised a myriad of practical treatment issues, not the least of which was the adoption of a useful model of true community care. As Dr. Freedman wrote [38, p. 183]:

> My unease is that we have not been able clearly to speak of mental health 'in' the community rather than community mental health centers as but one component or device to that end. We have been unable to get to new pragmatics of community health, since we must always connote new institutions with their credos and careers. . . . We are prisoners of programmatic needs and rhetoric and may lose sight of the patient who is our charge.

If a model of mental health in the community was lacking, so was the original political environment which informed NIMH's mission. Dr. Freedman wrote, "The agency became a prisoner of its constituencies, and responsibility for professionally accountable treatments received, of necessity, less emphasis or priority than did advocacy" [38, p. 187].

Ironically, perhaps it was the very lack of a unified and convincing model of community that lead to the rise of special interests within the fragmenting political and economic environment of the times. While mainstream mental illness professionals continued to be caught up in immediate issues of direct care to clients, public mental health planners continued to struggles over the meaning of community. The fatal flaw was, and continues to be in the 1990s, that such an entity may well not exist beyond the minds of mental health planners, professionals, and idealistic policymakers.

AFTERMATH
FROM CENTERS TO SYSTEMS AND BEYOND,
LATE 1970s TO 1990

The Carter Commission Report led to a change in the federal conceptualization of the CMHC program from community centers to mental health systems. The CMHC program was renamed The Community Support Program (CSP). Individual states were brought back into the planning and allocation process, and funding was focused away from the growth of comprehensive centers to the encouragement of systems of care. Systems of care were to serve the wide range of treatment populations addressed in the Presidential Commission's Report [39] and were to be networked in such a way as to ensure a smooth flow of patients among appropriate treatments. Special attention was paid to the chronically mentally ill—an emphasis that was to continue into the 1990s. The CSP plan had just gotten underway when the Carter Presidency ended and with it the legislative underpinning for CSPs.

Rosalyn Carter, the former first lady and one of the prime movers of the Administration's interest in mental health, continued to pursue her interests in improving care through conferences and initiatives sponsored by the Carter Center in Atlanta, Georgia. But this locally notable effort fell far short of the power and influence available to her and to CMHC policy makers during the Carter presidency.

FROM SYSTEMS TO BLOCK GRANTS, 1980 TO 1986

With the passing of the Carter Administration came the demise of executive support for categorical CMHC funding. The Reagan years were a time of diminished federal involvement and uneven state involvement in the politics and funding of mental illness treatment.

Under Reagan's Administration, states and localities were given direct control over decreasing federal mental health monies. CSP monies were replaced by the Reagan Block Grant Program. Funds which previously had been used for direct funding of individual federal programs were now pooled under the title of Block Grants. In 1981, mental health funds were lumped together with funds for a myriad programs and subsumed by the title, Alcohol, Drug Abuse, and Mental Health Block Grants. Federal monies were stepped down over four years with the expectation that states would pick up the difference for programs which were locally valued. This era was marked marked by intense infighting among agencies for the diminishing funds [40].

As of 1975, the United States Department of Health and Human Services (HHS) dropped from its data collection system the category of "federally funded community mental health centers" thereby marking in another way the official termination of federal involvement in the CMHC movement.

INPATIENT AND OUTPATIENT TREATMENT TRENDS

Despite the decrease in direct categorical funding for CMHC facilities during the 1980s, rates of admission to mental health facilities continued to climb. With the withdrawal of federal funding, general hospitals, private psychiatric facilities, and what Kiesler in

1980 called the *de facto* care system, including nursing homes, welfare hotels, prisons, and the streets grew in importance [41].

Due to the decrease in length of stay, and to the limitations imposed on treatment by third party payers, rates of treatment changed. Rates also changed as the availability of facilities reflected the withdrawal of public monies from inpatient institutions. Inpatient rates at state and county psychiatric hospitals fell steadily from 1975 to 1986, while inpatient rates at general hospitals and private psychiatric hospitals steadily increased, the latter by more than one-third between 1983 and 1986 [42]. This reflected the resolve on the part of most states to continue removing inpatient beds from state mental hospitals, a trend which had been at the heart of the move to deinstitutionalize. Unfortunately, this trend did not reflect the continuing lack of innovative community alternatives. Medicaid and private insurance coverage also limited and directed the flow of patients into non-institutionalized settings.

Rates of psychiatric outpatient admissions rose steadily from 1975 to 1986. Rates of outpatient treatment at state and county hospitals dropped sharply from 69 per 100,000 population in 1975 to 26 in 1986, again a reflection of state policies to cut back on state hospital care. Rates at general hospitals rose from 120 per 100,000 population in 1985 to 206 in 1986. At private psychiatric hospitals, the rates rose dramatically with the expansion of the for-profit sector. Rates rose from 16 per 100,000 in 1975 to 52 per 100,000 population in 1986 [42, p. 198].

Rates of admission to partial hospitalization programs fell markedly at state and county hospitals from 7 per 100,000 population in 1975 to 2 per 100,000 in 1986. Rates at such programs in general hospitals more than doubled in that time, as did rates for programs at private hospitals [42, p. 198].

The impact of the reduction of direct federal funding for community alternatives and the continued state insistence on deinstitutionalization was reflected not only in the rates and sites of treatment, but also in the rates of treatment by diagnosis. For examples, between 1975 and 1986, rates of inpatient admissions for alcoholism to state and county psychiatric facilities dropped from 50 per 100,000 population to 23. During that same time, alcohol admissions to general hospital psychiatric facilities rose from 17 per 100,000 to 41 per 100,000 population [42, p. 202].

Among other chronic disorders, schizophrenia for example, similar trends emerged. Admissions for schizophrenia dropped from 61 per 100,000 to 50 at state and county hospitals, while increasing slightly at general hospitals [42, p. 202]. The revolving door of admission, discharge, and readmission seemed to have replaced the long-term, custodial stay in state hospitals.

STAFFING TRENDS

An analysis of the reshuffling of full-time equivalent (FTE) patient care staff in mental health organizations from 1976 to 1986 reveals trends which paralleled the trends shifts in treatment sites.

According to federal statistics, state and county mental hospitals FTEs decreased by over 22,000 during the decade, declining from over 141,000 FTEs in 1976 to about 119,000 FTEs in 1986 [42, p. 210]. The two categories of employees with loses were psychiatrists, losing 571 FTEs, and the lowest paid workers, categorized as "other mental health workers," losing over 30,000 FTEs during the period. Despite the losses in this latter category, these employees continued to constitute more than half of the patient care personnel in state and county hospitals.

General hospital psychiatric services almost doubled FTEs in the same period from about 34,000 in 1976 to over 61,000 in 1986. The biggest gains came in nursing and "other professional staff" which gained about 32,000 FTEs. Psychiatry increased by over 2,000 FTEs. Here again, the lowest paid workers lost almost 2,000 FTEs, dropping from 38 percent of the staff to 18 percent [42, p. 210].

Private psychiatric hospitals also more than doubled their FTEs from about 17,000 in 1976 to over 35,000 in 1986. Again the biggest gains came in nursing, 6,5752 FTEs, and "other professional workers," to 7,323 FTEs. In these institutions, "other mental health workers" increased slightly. In terms of overall staffing for private psychiatric hospitals, "other mental health workers" fell from 43 percent of the total patient staff to 23 percent in 1986. These figures suggest a continuing trend toward rebuilding job tasks which had previously been divided among specialized categories of other workers. For example, nurses or other skilled workers would be expected to do the tasks formerly done by others yet would receive little or no additional pay compensation.

AN OVERVIEW OF PATTERNS, 1975 TO 1986

During this period private hospitals served as treatment centers for those with sufficient third-party payment while board-and-care homes, the street, welfare hotels or prisons may have served as "community" facilities for many of the rest. Exact figures are impossible to obtain, but according to Shadish, et al., HHS reported that as of the late 1970s, among residents of nursing homes, at least 30 percent suffered from a chronic mental disorder other than senility [43]. Shadish et al. noted that Medicaid regulations prohibited more than 50 percent of nursing home residents to have a primary diagnosis of mental illness, thereby potentially leading to under reporting of such diagnoses [43, p. 3].

These same authors estimated that an additional 400,000 chronic mental patients resided in board-and-care homes in the early 1980s, with the remaining patients scattered across many other settings. Only 15 percent were estimated to be in mental hospitals at any one time.

With the withdrawal of federal funds, much of the political impetus for supporting mental illness care returned to individual states. In 1987 the State Commissioner of the Oklahoma Department of Mental Health, J. Frank James, answered the question: "Does the Community Mental Health Movement Have the Momentum Needed to Survive?" [44]. The answer he felt was yes. In support of his answer, the Commissioner cited examples of states which continued to focus on providing non-institutionalized care for the chronically mentally ill, on NIMH's continued support for alternative care, and on lobbying by such groups as the National Alliance for the Mentally Ill on behalf of expanded noninstitutionalized care. The author admitted that, "It is true that some states proceeded with removing patients from hospitals without regard for need or resources available. To be simplistic, California, for example, removed the funds and left the patients; New York removed the patients and left the funds" [44, p. 449]. But the author's pessimism was offset by his review of data contained in a 1985 survey of state mental health commissioners who overwhelmingly reported no trend toward re-institutionalization yet no reduction of screening or aftercare due to budget cutting [44, p. 449]. It is perhaps not unexpected that state commissioners would be reluctant to admit declining quality of care during their own terms of office.

As with health care in general [45] by the end of the 1980s, psychiatric patients and service providers were facing a non-system of services heavy laden with concerns over costs and output. As usually, clinicians and politicians saw the problems differently. In a telling 1990 editorial in the *American Journal of Orthopsychiatry*, Matthew Dumont the Medical Director of a community counseling center, wrote [46, p. 167]:

> Managed mental health care, seen against the background of the community mental health movement, is merely the commodification of caring, the transformation of treatment into business and the exploitation of professionalism. It is consistent with these decadent and kindless times.

In sum the removal of federal funding for CMHCs and mental health systems during the 1980s had, to a significant degree, left a void of responsibility for overall care planning and implementation. Most states continued to withdraw support form state psychiatric facilities while doing relatively little in terms of replacing beds with permanent community based alternatives. Largely as a result, general hospital psychiatric unites and private psychiatric hospitals had moved to the center of the treatment arena. Care, perhaps now more than ever since the inception of the CMHC movement, depended importantly on the patient's ability to pay and to negotiate through the nonsystem of services. Those with poor or no payment source might end up in the *de facto* system, receiving custodial care with minimal or no active treatment. Those with good payment sources might choose among a rich variety of treatment sites in the fast expanding for-profit sector.

A BRIEF LOOK AT THEORY IN THE CMHC MOVEMENT'S AFTERMATH

With the demise of the movement came a significant decline in the theoretical exploration of community in the literature. Rather than argue over the meaning of community, authors now argued over what it all had signified or over which state was doing the best job for its ex-patients. Many, looking back over the movement which had been heralded as a revolution several decades earlier, now saw a crazy quilt pattern of charges and counter-charges about the very meaning of mental illness.

Although patterns of theory were fragmented, certain competing themes did emerge: 1) elaboration of a model of mental illness which focused on the unity of mind and body thus reaffirming the medical/ psychiatric role as the primary source for mental illness treatment; 2) psychiatric nihilism; and 3) reduction of issues of community to issues of ethics and law.

Roth and Kroll in their work, *The Reality of Mental Illness*, reflected two of these themes, i.e. reaffirmation of the medical model and reduction of issues to legal considerations [47]. The tone and content were consensual but were so in a somewhat defensive voice as if responding to the earlier critics. Wrote Roth and Kroll [47, p. 45]:

> For some critics of capitalist society, it is convenient to blame the evils of capitalism for the existence of mental illness. But such a standpoint must be rooted strictly in an environmental theory of causation which ignores the contribution of genetics, metabolic abnormalities, and even biological variability and vulnerability. That such theoretical gymnastics are not inherent in the nature of Marxist reasoning is clear from the concept of mental illness in contemporary China. There, dialectical materialism prevails but the environment is not blamed for the occurrence of mental illness.

This suggested a lack of understanding of the history of Chinese psychiatry. (See discussion of this in Chapter 6.) The extent of amnesia related to the previous decade's romance with the P.R.C. is nicely reflected in the statement that Chinese society is uniformly characterized by dialectical materialism—a highly questionable charge, even if a definition of the concept were given. More important to the current analysis is the lack of recognition of the multi-varied conflict themes which had emerged during the middle phase of the CMHC movement. In the late 1960s and early 1970s, authors were articulating not one attack on psychiatry from one Marxist perspective, but many attacks from many neo-marxist perspectives. (See Chapter 6.)

Another unfortunate implication of the author's words was the lack of historical insight brought to the charge that Chinese psychiatry failed to blame the environment for mental illness. Indeed, concepts of the environment had been central to indigenous cultural under-standings of mental illness in China for centuries, and specific maoist-marxist interpretations came to particular prominence in psychiatric treatment during the 1970s.

A somewhat surprising entry into the camp of those who reaffirmed the need for a stronger psychiatric presence in addressing the problem was E. Fuller Torrey, a prominent voice against the medical model of psychiatry in the 1970s. In his 1974 book, *The Death of Psychiatry*, Dr. Torrey had written [48, p. 194]:

> I have said that the medical model of human behavior should be banished to the realm of the dodo bird and the dinosaur. When its medical rhetoric is followed to its logical conclusion, it ends up in the land of the absurd. . . . In place of the medical model, I have

proposed an educational model. . . . The boundaries between psychiatry, psychology, anthropology, sociology, and the other artificial disciplines would be abolished as would the disciplines themselves. Present practitioners of these disciplines would become behavioral scientists and in the case of psychiatry some would return to being neurologists.

By 1988 in his volume, *Nowhere to Go: The Tragic Odyssey of the Homeless Mentally Ill* Dr. Torrey was calling for psychiatric professionals to be required by each state to provide four hours a month of free service to the seriously mentally ill or lose their licenses to practice [49]. The author mentioned several organizations as potentially providing leadership for this and other service reforms. He wrote of his hope in the National Alliance for the Mentally Ill and the National Mental Health Consumers Association to mobilize their energies and push for reform. As organizations made up of patients and patient's families, he felt these, in concert with concerned providers, could form the core of a strong new mental health lobby. Still, the emphasis was returned to the sphere of psychiatric practice.

In addition to theorists who had returned to the medical/psychiatric emphasis, many authors have preferred to focus on the ethical and legal issues rather than on social theoretical issues within the literature. Confining the arena of discourse to ethics and the law allowed authors to address injustices without straying into the dangerous territory of conflict analysis or the larger political economic context [50]. Policy implications centered on use or reform of the legal system rather than on outright class struggle.

Authors into the early 1980s echoed the humanist conflict tone of anti-psychiatry activists in the 1960s and 1970s. Such groups as the Metal Patients Liberation Project in New York and the Coalition Against Forced Treatment in San Francisco, spent considerable energy writing about the possible empowerment of expsychiatric "inmates." An interesting example was *Madness Network News*, published during the late 1970s and the early 1980s by activists in San Francisco. The paper frequently published angry pieces by ex-mental patients who had experienced involuntary commitment or who had received unwanted drugs or other treatment.

But these earlier cries for reform and justice took on rather different implications in the mid-to-late 1980s when calls for reform were authored by "experts" for audiences of psychiatrists, hospital administrators, the police and other agents of social control. Stories of searches for personal liberation turned to tomes on institutional liability.

The decade of the 1980s had also brought with it voices of total psychiatric nihilism ringing with the rage of the 1960s and 1970s but without the theoretical underpinnings to point a way out of the morass. These authors conveyed a sense that the whole matter was hopeless, that both legitimated psychiatric care givers and their critics were unwittingly intertwined in an exercise in futility. Such a work was well represented by Masson's *Against Therapy: Emotional Tyranny and the Myth of Psychological Healing* [51]. Here the author attacked what he called those who profited off another's misery. Freud, Jung, the humanists, and feminists were all equally at fault for profiting economically from their patients and for accepting existing therapeutic standards which dehumanized the individual. A variation on this theme, which seemed to be emerging by the end of the decade, was the call for a return to the ideal of self-help, a theme which served both traditional voluntary organizations such as The National Association for the Mentally Ill as well as offshoots from anti-psychiatry.

In sum, the aftermath of the movement left disenchantment and distrust among many. The failure of the search for community breed a return to faith only in the reality of the individual standing alone.

REFERENCES

1. H. Freed, Promoting Accountability in Mental Health Services: The Negotiated Mandate, *American Journal of Orthopsychiatry, 42*, pp. 253-254, 1972.
2. S. Schifff, Community Accountability and Mental Health Services, *Mental Hygiene, 54*, pp. 205-214, 1970.
3. United States Congress, *Federal Register, 37*:28, 1972.
4. F. D. Chu and S. Trotter, *The Madness Establishment*, Grossman Publishing, New York, 1974.
5. B. L. Bloom, *Community Mental Health: A General Introduction*, Brooks/Cole Publishing, Montery, California, 1977.
6. J. W. Lounsbury, K. G. Roeseim, L. Pokorny, A. Sills, and G. J. Neissen, An Analysis of Topic Areas and Topic Trends in the *Community Mental Health Journal*, from 1965 through 1977, *Community Mental Health Journal, 15*, pp. 267-276, 1979.
7. P. M. Roman and H. Trice (eds.) *Sociological Perspectives on Community Mental Health*, F. A. Davis, Philadelphia, 1974.

8. J. D. Preston, The Meaning of 'Community' in Community Psychiatry, in *Sociological Perspectives on Community Mental Health*, P. Roman and H. Trice (eds.), F. A. Davis, Philadelphia, pp. 51-67, 1974.

9. K. P. Wilkinson, The Community as a Social Field, *Social Forces, 48*, pp. 311-322, 1970.

10. W. H. Dunham, Community Psychiatry: The Newest Therapeutic Bandwagon, *Archives of General Psychiatry*, pp. 303-313, 1965.

11. H. Dunham, *Social Realities and Community Psychiatry*, Behavioral Publications, New York, 1976.

12. A. J. Nassi, Community Control or Control of the Community?: The Case of the Community Mental Health Center, *Journal of Community Psychology*, 6, pp. 3-15, 1978.

13. D. C. Klein, Some Reflections on Community Control: A Commentary on Nassi, *Journal of Community Psychology*, 6, pp. 16-18, 1978.

14. P. R. Dokecki, A Transactional Perspective on the Interrelationship of the Societal Power Structure, the Mental Health Establishment, the Individual, and the Community: A Commentary on Nassi, *Journal of Community Psychology*, 6, pp. 19-21, 1978.

15. K. H. Flaming, Community Control in a Gesellschaft World: A Comment, *Journal of Community Psychology*, 6, pp. 22-24, 1978.

16. S. Bernstein, L. Cooper, E. Currie, J. Frappis, S. Harring, T. Platt, P. Poyner, G. Ray, J. Scruggs, and L. Trijillo, *The Iron Fist in the Velvet Glove: An Analysis of the U.S. Police*, Center for Research on Criminal Justice, Berkeley, California, 1977.

17. L. Bellak, *A Concise Handbook of Community Psychiatry and Community Mental Health*, Grune and Stratton, New York, 1974.

18. W. Bolman, Policy Aspects of Citizen Participation, in *A Concise Handbook of Community Psychiatry and Community Mental Health*, L. Bellak (ed.), Grune and Stratton, New York, pp. 219-241, 1974.

19. D. C. Regester, Community Mental Health—For Whose Community? *American Journal of Public Health*, 9, pp. 886-893, 1974.

20. F. U. Mannino, B. Maclenna, M. F. Shore (eds.), *The Practice of Mental Health Consultation*, Gardner Press, New York, 1975.

21. S. C. Plog and P. I. Ahmed, *Principles and Techniques of Mental Health Consultation*, Plenum Medical Book Company, New York, 1977.

22. M. S. Gibbs, J. R. Lachenmeyer, and J. Sigal (eds.) *Community Psychology: Theoretical and Empirical, Approaches*, Gardner Press, New York, 1980.

23. K. Heller and J. Monahan, *Psychology and Community Change*, The Dorsey Press, Homewood, Illinois, 1977.

24. P. A. Mann, *Community Psychology: Concepts and Application*, The Free Press, New York, 1978.

25. J. Zusman and C. R. Wurster, *Program Evaluation: Alcohol, Drug Abuse and Mental Health Services*, Lexington Books, Lexington, Massachusetts, 1975.

26. J. Morrison and M. Sundel, Development of a Community Assessment Strategy for Program Evaluation in a Comprehensive Human Service Delivery System, in *Program Evaluation: Alcohol, Drug Abuse, and Mental Health Services*, J. Zusman and C. R. Wurster (eds.), Lexington Books, Lexington, Massachusetts, pp. 161-170, 1975.

27. D. C. Riedel, G. L. Tishler, and J. K. Myers, *Patient Care Evaluation in Mental Health Programs*, Ballinger Publishing, Cambridge, Massachusetts, 1974.

28. G. L. Tishler, J. Henisz, J. K. Myers, and P. Boswell, Utilization of Mental Health Services, *Archives of General Psychiatry*, *32*, pp. 411-415, 1975.

29. B. L. Bloom, *Changing Patterns of Psychiatric Care*, Behavioral Publications, New York, 1975.

30. E. W. Markson and D. F. Allen (eds.), *Trends in Mental Health Evaluation*, Lexington Books, Lexington, Massachusetts, 1975.

31. I. Davidoff, M. Guttentag, and J. Offrett (eds.), *Evaluating Community Mental Health Services*, U.S. Dept. of H.E.W., Washington, D.C., 1977.

32. R. A. Dorwart and W. R. Meyers, *Citizen Participation in Mental Health: Research and Social Policy*, Charles C. Thomas Publisher, Springfield, Illinois, 1981.

33. C. C. Attkisson, W. A. Hargreaves, and J. E. Sorensen, *Evaluation of Human Service Programs*, Academic Press, New York, 1978.

34. H. Hafner, *Estimating Needs for Mental Health Policy*, Springer-Verlag, New York, 1979.

35. E. J. Posavac (ed.), *Impacts of Program Evaluation on Mental Health Care*, Westview Press, Boulder, Colorado, 1977.

36. J. P. Brady and H. K. Brodie (eds.), *Psychiatry at the Crossroads*, The Saunders Press, Philadelphia, 1978.

37. President's Commission on Mental Health, *Report to the President's Commission on Mental Health*, U.S. Government Printing Office, Washington, D.C., 1978.

38. D. X. Freedman, Community Mental Health: Slogan or New Direction?, in *Psychiatry at the Crossroads*, J. P. Brady and H. K. Brodie (eds.), The Saunders Press, Philadelphia, pp. 179-189, 1978.

39. J. P. Morrissey and H. G. Goldman, Cycles of Reform in the Care of the Chronically Mentally Ill, *Hospital and Community Psychiatry*, *35*, pp. 785-793, 1984.

40. A. B. Johnson, *Out of Bedlam: The Truth about Deinstitutionalization*, Basic Books, New York, 1990.

41. C. A. Kiesler, Mental Health Policy as a Field of Inquiry, *American Psychologist*, *35*, pp. 1066-1080, 1980.

42. U.S. Department of Health and Human Services, National Center for Health Statistics, *Health*, Public Health Service, Hyattsville, Maryland, 1989.

43. W. R. Shadish, Jr., A. J. Lurigio, and D. A. Lewis, After Deinstitutionalization: The Present and Future of Mental Health Long-Term Care Policy,
Journal of Social Issues, 45, 1-15, 1989.
44. J. F. James, Does the Community Mental Health Movement Have the
Momentum Needed to Survive?, *American Journal of Orthopsychiatry, 57*,
pp. 447-451, 1987.
45. R. H. Elling, The Fiscal Crisis of the State and State Financing of Health
Care—Toward a Conceptual and Action Statement for Improved Public
Support of Medical and Health Care, *Social Science and Medicine, 15C*,
pp. 207-217, 1981.
46. M. Dumont, Managed Care, Managed People, and Community Mental
Health, *American Journal of Orthopsychiatry, 60*, pp. 166-167, 1990.
47. M. Roth and J. Kroll, *The Reality of Mental Illness*, Cambridge University
Press, Cambridge, 1986.
48. E. F. Torrey, *The Death of Psychiatry*, Penguin Books, New York, 1974.
49. E. F. Torrey, *Nowhere to Go: The Tragic Odyssey of the Homeless Mentally
Ill*, Harper & Row, New York, 1988.
50. R. Isaac and V. C. Armat, *Madness in the Street: How Psychiatry and the
Law Abandoned the Mentally Ill*, The Free Press, New York, 1990.
51. J. M. Masson, *Against Therapy: Emotional Tyranny and the Myth of
Psychological Healing*, Athenaeum, New York, 1988.

CHAPTER 8

Conclusions toward a Sociology of Applied Sociology

The CMHC movement had been heralded as a revolution by its founders. Many had envisioned the movement as producing a rational system of care, one which moved away from psychoanalytic psychotherapy for the wealthy and custodial care in large state institutions for the poor. Many movement participants hoped for an organized network of care givers, situated in communities across the United States, who would be able to provide basic help at that local level for all clients, but who also would be ready and able appropriately to refer clients to more specialized treatment when necessary. A public health approach, that is one which situated individual presentation of symptomatology in a larger socio-economic and cultural context, was adopted as the basis for much of the CMHC rhetoric.

Yet saying this is hardly new. What is new is the realization of just how broad and varied the CMHC visions proved to be. CMHC participants transformed what at first seemed to be one model into a succession of models, each reflecting the immediate concerns of administrators, staff, and funders. During particularly active periods, patients and patient advocates also made their voices heard in the streets and in the movement literature. All of their models reflected the dynamics of federal mental health policies, of the mental illness treatment marketplace, and of worldwide political and economic forces.

In this concluding chapter a summary of these political and economic influences is presented. An overview of State, market, and theory is summarized and explored. Works of sociologists of knowledge are addressed, and suggestions for the answering of the title questions, i.g. Who plays? Who pays?, and Who cares? are given.

Table 9 summarizes the gist of the preceding analysis. It shows that as economic periods emerged and receded, the concept of community changed in parallel fashion.

During the era of the 1950s and early 1960s, public health psychiatry at the federal level flourished under the influence of key psychiatrists and federal legislators. The vision of community mental health centers during this period was one of community workshops for public health psychiatrists. The community was defined as the pool of potential psychiatric patients. In the initial CMHC regulations, this vision was transformed into the pragmatics of catchmenting—dividing geographic areas into planning regions. Psychiatrists at these centers were envisioned as not only treating patients through conventional therapeutic interventions, but as providing outreach in the form of consultation and education. CMHC workers would consult to community leaders, teaching them techniques of primary prevention in order to stop mental health problems before they started. CMHC workers also were seen as educating the population in each catchment area about mental illness and improving early diagnosis and referral. Patients, it was believed, would be treated in their immediate geographic area and their therapy would not be dependent on ability to pay. Follow-up would be locally available and mental health workers would understand the social and cultural milieu in which patients functioned on a daily basis. All of this was mirrored in the seemingly simple term "community."

By the mid to late 1960s it became clear that the centers would not be staffed primarily by psychiatrists, let alone psychiatrists trained in public health psychiatry. There weren't enough to go around, and many psychiatrists preferred other practice settings. A multitude of provider groups came flooding into the provider slots established by and funded through federal CMHC monies. Social workers, nurses, psychologists, and others made the centers home for their work and for their visions of mental health practice. They brought with them, into the professional CMHC literature, new visions and new rhetorics of community. The consensual view of community as psychiatrist's workplace was replaced with ardent cries that community existed wherever workers fought bosses, minorities fought racists, feminists fought sexists, or

Table 9. Summary of State, Market, and Theory during the Three Major Phases of the Community Mental Health Movement

Period	Market Trends	State Functions	Legislation and Regulations	Concept of Community
Period I: late 1950s to mid 1960s	Market infrastructure expanded through federal monies. Monopoloy sector in control.	Accumulated surplus expended. Force targeted at urban areas. Mental health and social services seen as ideological control.	Initial CMHC legislations and regulations passed. Five services are mandated.	Community = catchment area, doctors' service area, consensual field/system.
Period II: mid 1960s to early 1970s	Infrastructure expansion continues with federal monies. Division of labor articulated. Competitive sector drawn into market.	Force widened to more diverse groups. Factions form around traditionalists and "radicals."	CMHC legislation renewed with expanded funding. Children and addicts added as target patient populations.	Community = value consensus versus Community = class struggle
Period III: early 1970s to 1980	Market stabilizes. Funding emphasis switched to states and private sector.	Political support weakens. Special interest groups consolidate lobbying.	New planning schemes define consumers and providers. Evaluation emphasized. Carter administration produce President's Commission Report and Mental Health Systems Act.	Community = consensual field, Gemeinschaft, consensual interest groups, networks of services
Aftermath 1980 to 1990	Market fragments into public and private, good and poor payment sources.	Impetus returned to state governments and private sector.	Reagan block grants replace CMHC funding. Most federal money withdrawn.	Community largely disappears from literature.

199

where mental patients/ prisoners fought their therapists/subjugators. Community became a field of conflict.

In response, the more conservative elements in the movement countered that community was not a battlefield. Community was an ordered, structured grouping of the populace. Community had leaders and followers. Community had legitimate authorities who had the skill and knowledge necessary to help the mentally ill. This was the community that was to be served calmly and professionally by the CMHC workers.

By the early 1970s, again the federal political winds shifted and funding became increasingly contested. Just as the CMHC rhetoric reached new peaks of ferocity in the literature, the ground rules changed. The goal was no longer to define which provider group could be considered more knowledgeable and powerful than another, but to define who could show need for service, and to prove who could best meet that need. Evaluation and accountability ruled the day.

By the mid 1970s, centers had become so unwieldy, suffering under the weight of more than ten mandated services, that they were legislatively transformed into systems. Mental health systems were to serve mental health consumer groups through the services of mental health providers. Authors spent a considerable amount of time drawing up detailed lists of providers and consumers and their duties.

By the late 1980s much of the CMHC movement had been erased. What had taken at least four decades to build, took only about four years to dismantle. With the end of federal funding came the end of the CMHC era. While a few hearty souls continued to debate what had happened with the federally financed CMHCs over the past decades, most turned instead to state-level initiatives and local model programs.

LESSONS IN THE SOCIOLOGY OF APPLIED SOCIOLOGY

What does all of this mean for understanding how social theory is applied outside of the discipline of sociology? The works of forebears of the sociology of knowledge are viewed here in search of answers.

Marx and Mannheim

A century and a half ago Marx argued that the ruling ideas of an age were the ideas of the rulers. Mannheim elaborated on this general theme by asserting that intellectuals were not truly members of one class but acted instead as satellites of one or another existing class.

The authors who created the CMHC literature could not be considered members of one class. They represented many occupational and professional groups as well as diverse theoretical perspectives. Interestingly authors within any one profession often represented opposing views within that profession. Leftists and conservatives, conflict theorists and consensualists, priests and prophets, could all be found within the profession of medicine. Likewise, scholars representing all these traditions were found throughout disciplines associated with the movement. It did seem that psychologists felt more at ease with the concept of community than did psychiatrists, and that they took conflict theory more to heart. But during the flowering of conflict theory, even elite psychiatric journals and staunch supporters of consensualism, grudgingly acknowledged the existence of the issues raised by conflict analysis.

It seems from this particular study that priestly and prophetic scholars were not so much representing class differences as they were their own intellectual inclinations. It is clear that voices of what started as a minority tradition flourished when historical circumstances allowed development of critical masses of prophetic scholars sharing their ideas. When enough voices were heard repeating nontraditional ideas, then lines of communication began to emerge among authors and an audience became defined. It was not the case that the intuitive correctness or intellectual merits of these nontraditional ideas were enough to gain them standing within the professional literature. What was needed was activist support from a significant number of like-minded individuals, along with political and economic conditions which supported change in the larger society. Whether or not conflict theory, an alternative theoretical tradition could be conceptualized as a unified class culture is highly questionable. But it is clear that when historical circumstances favored consolidation of this non-traditional view, it did find a place within the professional literature of the CMHC movement.

This case study did support Mannheim's concept of the importance of social generation. It was the case that scholars and activists who experienced the same historical conditions did react to them in somewhat similar ways, at least they were more likely to frame their analyses in similar fashions. In the middle years of the movement, conflict authors reacted against consensual definitions of the situation and consensualists reacted to conflict rhetoric. In the ending phase of the movement, the definition changed to reflect the emerge of interest groups and the language which accompanied their growth. Another lesson to be learned from this is that no single social theory, when applied outside the discipline, can be totally dominant in the literature. A balance exists—often a balance heavily tipped toward theories which serve dominant political and economic interests, but nonetheless a balance. Control of the literature by one particular group is never total. Nor is socialization to a particular profession or occupation enough to explain the adoption of a particular set of sociological background assumptions. When and how the balance between theories changes depends significantly on the external politics and economics in the larger society rather than on the creations of professional scholars. In sum, it does not seem that the ruling ideas are the ideas of the rulers. It seems rather that within the ruling ideas there are dominant and non-dominant themes which emerge and recede as historical conditions nudge them first one way then another.

Gramsci

Gramsci had elaborated on Marx by suggesting that sets of ideas were not mirror reflections of some deeper political economic infrastructure or of classes. Gramsci felt that ideas could be seen as somewhat autonomous from market and State forces, and at times the ideas themselves could influence the course of political economic struggle. In this sense culture became a primary factor in class conflict.

Gramsci described the slow and tortuous emergence of what he saw as liberated organic ideologies, i.e. sets of ideas which reflected liberated views of life. Gramsci felt that these ideologies were created through consciously organizing the understandings of everyday life, especially through organizing the understandings of struggles related to economic and political hardship or turmoil.

According to this way of thinking, scholars ought to be connected to the daily struggles of ordinary people in order to add their expertise to the development of liberated ideologies. Through developing liberated culture within journalism, art, literature, and scholarly work, scholars could help to make everyday life coherent and understandable to those who sought such understandings. These scholars could build a basis for a scholarship and for a culture which helped to free the ordinary person from the clutch of exploitative, taken-for-granted understandings of the self and of the world.

It might be argued that conflict scholarship and political activism in the late 1960s and early 1970s provided this rather special connection between scholarship and daily struggle. Indeed many of the conflict scholars whose work was influential during this period had personally experienced the battles at Lincoln Hospital or elsewhere between "professionals" and "the community". Their experience was mirrored in both the tone and content of their scholarship. The overtly emotional tone which marked their works frequently echoed events from the streets or wards.

But the works of these authors were not distinctive because they had somehow escaped their class linkages or overcome their professional socialization, as Gramsci might have argued. Instead, scholars had found room or made room within their disciplines in order to voice their scholarship. Psychiatrists didn't stop practicing psychiatry, they started practicing radical psychiatry. Likewise social workers, and others often stayed within their occupations or professions while creating new practice modalities.

Gramsci may have been partially correct in describing the emergence of organic ideology as a slow process. But the case of the CMHC literature suggests that alternatives are continuously emerging. They break through into mainstream thought when the political and economic conditions favor a shift in the balance between the priests and prophets, between those who accept the essentials of the given social structure and those who would replace them.

At what point a prophetic theory becomes complete enough or strong enough to challenge a dominant priestly view is an empty question without specific historical referents. Abstracting theory from its historical context becomes an exercise in mental gymnastics, rather devoid of meaning for those who seek to understand how and why theories change.

Another important point related to the Gramscian concept of organic ideologies is that scholarship can emerge from many occupational and professional spheres to serve either dominant or non-dominant views. It is not so much the discipline which determines the language of theory, but it is theory which reflects ideological schools cutting across disciplines. Unlike those who would argue that the theory of a discipline is applied primarily in service of that discipline, this study has suggested that one theory can be applied by various authors for varying needs. For example, consensual theory served planners, clinicians, politicians, and administrators.

This study also has suggested that conflict theory with its accompanying ideological implications can be produced by scholars who themselves are members of an elite professional group. In some cases it may be that publication of such alternative approaches may actually enhance the dominant factions by providing a sense of intellectual democracy within a professional literature without truly swaying readers through force of reason or logic. In the end, perhaps the central Gramscian question remains whether theory qua ideology is a reflection of larger market and State forces or is itself a semi-autonomous creation by liberated scholars? This study suggests that emphasis rests more certainly on the macro-structural forces.

Friedrichs and Gouldner

Both Friedrichs and Gouldner voiced a plea to scholars to look inward during the process of theorizing. They urged scholars to reflect on their works with a heightened sensitivity as to their personal assumptions and ideological orientations. Both authors seemed to feel that authentic attempts at self-awareness could provide intellectuals with a means to escape the hold of political and economic forces. Gouldner termed this process reflexive sociology: Friedrich conceptualized the process as witnessing or engaging in dialectical dialogue.

As concerns the authors and works surveyed in the case of the CMHC literature, there seems little evidence that such self-awareness or good-faith dialogue swayed authors from one or another point of view. Consensualists remained consensualists, albeit modifying their brand of consensualism as the focus of debate shifted. Conflict theorist remained conflict theorist though they also modified their brand of conflict as themes in the literature and in their private lives emerged and disappeared. Although some anti-psychiatry authors have left potent impressions of soul-searching through the track of their written words, there is little reason to believe that staunch consensualists were any less self-aware or sincere. And there is little evidence here to lend support to the argument that reflexive insights or open dialogue convinced authors to change theoretical camps.

Lee

Perhaps Alfred McClung Lee came closest to offering applied scholars a way to gain conscious control over their products. In his *Sociology for Whom* Lee remained scholars of the necessity to produce their work within a collectivity of like-minded individuals, to criticize abuses within one's own discipline, and to focus attention on the public manipulation of scholarly works [1]. It is certainly the case that scholars working within applied fields need to be sensitized to the uses to which their work is put in professional applications and in the public consciousness. The public's interpretation of scholarship can redefine meanings so that what might start as an intra-professional dialogue becomes a street fight among bystanders.

In the end, often regardless of the personal intentions of an author, once words are put forth for public consumption, the author's control is lost. This point was forcefully illustrated by Spector and Kitsuse in their analysis of changing definitions of social problems [2]. As they documented in their case of the political uses of Soviet psychiatry (see Chapter 2 for a more detailed description), definitions of "problems" can rise and fall as inter-professional rivalries proceed, as audiences for scholarly works change, and as political contexts change. What might begin as well-meaning cooperation can turn rather subtly to dissent.

WHO PLAYS?, WHO PAYS?, WHO CARES?

The first chapter ended with the posing of three basic questions related to the understanding of applied scholarship, i.e. Who plays?, Who pays?, Who cares? It is through answers to these questions that a systematic understanding can be gained of how and why social theory is applied outside of sociology.

Who Plays?

The players in the CMHC movement included social scientists, planners, clinicians, politicians, administrators, mental patients, patient advocates, and a host of others. Some held exceedingly traditional views, what Friedrichs termed priestly outlooks on the world. A certain segment of these began their participation in the movement believing that it would usher in a new age of humanitarian mental illness treatment. Four decades later their enthusiasm seems misplaced. But in their roles they carried out their own brand of social engineering, a type of reformism born of their times and their professional socialization.

The prophetic players armed themselves with the rhetoric of righteousness. They fought hard, often on the front lines of street demonstrations as well as in the pages of professional works, They too urged their listeners on to the creation of a newly just society and a newly humane treatment model. Looking back now, they seem oddly naive.

Who Pays?

In answer to the first question, the answer was that both priests and prophets "played." Priests brought to their tasks the background assumptions of priests and they remained priests despite having to respond to prophets as their voices grew louder. Prophets likewise held steady to their theoretical orientations. But how were these authors funded during the shifting political economic context of the movement?

The answer was often that the federal government paid, at least during the first two phases of the movement. But in the later phase, as the government began to stabilize its funding and then withdraw funds, privatized profits became more highly prized by those on the receiving end. When the market consolidation was well underway and the political atmosphere had cooled from the activism and rhetoric of the 1960s, prophets lost funding outside certain university departments and thereby lost their room to maneuver as activists beyond the traditional scholarly setting. As their funded projects were reduced, their community of like-minded individuals began to wither and contract. With this came the disappearance of the prophetic themes in the CMHC literature. Some CMHC activists became tenured, secure "old-leftists" within the realm of academe, a fate shared by other prophet radicals of the times [3].[1] Others, like Michael Glenn, left the practice of psychiatry and broadened their scope—in Glenn's case by becoming a family practitioner.

The lack of wide state-level funding had considerable influence on the direction of the movement and ultimately on the literature. Seemingly the reason for this bypassing of the states was that local political interests feared enfranchisement of devalued groups. Local political powers were often beholden to those who hadn't shown a desire to fund or otherwise support CMHCs in particular neighborhoods. In fact, some feared that spending monies on devalued groups might empower them in ways which would fundamentally shift the local balance of political power. It was felt that a federal initiative might be able to bypass such local opposition and would be able to create centers without having to painfully negotiate with embedded local interests.

On the other hand, as Scull and others argued, it may well have been that a latent function served by CMHC funding was the shifting of costs from state institutions to the federal government [4]. Rather

---

[1] The impact of such tenured activists is the subject of heated debate. See for example the work of Roger Kimball.

than using state monies to support costly institutional care, federal monies were spent in support of social welfare, custodial homes, or the prison system.

As discussed in Chapter 4, during the early phase of the movement, the federal government had socialized the costs of the mental illness treatment market with significant profits fed back to the monopoly sector. In the second phase of the movement, the costs of the expanding market importantly included socializing the costs of the rapidly growing division of labor tied to CMHC care. The third phase of the movement was marked by a stabilization and then a diminishing of direct federal support. The expectation became one of shifting costs back to the monopoly sector. By the 1990s, private for-profit hospitals were absoring much of the profit. Publically funded hospitals and the ad hoc custodial system of the streets, welfare hotels, and prisons was incurring the expenses of housing former mental patients.

Who Cares?

The audience for the movement and for the movement's literature also clearly changed in line with political economic phases. As psychiatrists were replaced by social workers, psychologists, and others, a shifting series of themes attracted differing audiences.

Scholars who attempted to move into innovative applied roles within the activist movements found that they had to answer to persons who had guided scholarly production over the preceding decades. More senior consensual colleagues sat in judgement over their junior colleagues and often found little scholarly value in non-traditional activities [5].

Books which earlier might have been published by radical presses, by the 1980s and 1990s were now going wanting for publication either as those presses folded or were absorbed by other publishers. Journals which once published conflict works reflected the times by returning to variations on the consensual themes. Others such as *The Radical Therapist* appeared and disappeared rather quickly as the 1970s turned into the 1980s and conflict turned into quiescence.

Perhaps a word should be said here about modern sociologists of culture who explore these issues in relationship to scholarly production. Theorists such as Raymond Williams include in their analyses the impact of new technologies in reaching broader audiences and in forming new social contexts for discourse and organization around that discourse [6]. It is beyond the scope of the present work to take this particular issue beyond the CMHC movement, but within the movement, as has been shown here, traditional professional journals and texts did incorporate both prophetic and priestly voices in accord with the historical times.

How might younger participants in similar movements escape some of the pitfalls of the past, as least as they may be identified through this case study? First, applied social and behavioral scientists, both prophets and priests, should work, as Lee has suggested, within a community of like-minded individuals to the extent possible. In this way priestly peers may stand in judgement over priests; prophetic peers over prophets. Second, such persons may have to work on a series of short-term applied actions which, when taken in full, add to a fuller understanding of a basic issue in the scholarly discipline. Scholarly production may then be seen as a series of time-limited projects, often associated with applications outside of one's own discipline, but ones which systematically address discipline-specific issues.

An applied scholar of this sort might have to learn to be comfortable with the taking on of a variety of applied roles. At one point in time, such persons may have to be content with being passive observers. Direct action may have to wait. Always, such scholars must learn to chose their actions with great care, defining themselves to appropriate publics and advertising their skills to those they wish to serve.

Such applied scholars must maintain a delicate balance between the role of insider within a discipline and outsider. If they lose their scholarly identities, undoubtedly professional sanctions will be forthcoming. Promotion may be deferred or tenure refused.

For prophets, the case of the CMHC movement has pointed to the need to join thought with action as orthodox prophets have always preached. It may be that applied scholars in the late 1960s and early 1970s lost promising chances for far-reaching change by failing to have at their command the tools and tactics which had successfully served the priests. For example, it may be that rhetoric could have been transformed in ways which would have made them accessible to larger audiences. As this study has suggested, theoretical and ideological dominance is never complete but is a delicate balance between and among schools of thought. In these insights may be found fuller understanding of applications of theory beyond discipline-specific limitations.

REFERENCES

1. A. M-C. Lee, *Sociology for Whom?*, Oxford Press, New York, 1978.
2. M. Spector and J. I. Kitsuse, *Constructing Social Problems*, Aldine de Gruyter, New York, 1987.
3. R. Kimball, *Tenured Radicals: How Politics Has Corrupted Our Higher Education*, Harper & Row, New York, 1990.
4. A. T. Scull, *Decarceration*, Prentice Hall, Englewood Cliffs, New Jersey, 1977.
5. J. M. Wiener, Radical Historians and the Crisis in American History, 1959-1980, *The Journal of American History*, 76, pp. 339-435, 1989.
6. R. Williams, *Resources of Hope: Culture, Democracy, Socialism*, R. Gable (ed.), Verso, London, 1989.

APPENDIX

Methodology

SOURCES OF INFORMATION

Qualitative techniques including analysis of archival data and interviews were the chief data gathering tools for this research. Sources of data used in construction of the ideal types of theory, and those used in the analysis of the literature, were drawn from books and journals found in numerous libraries and four on-line searches. A wide variety of libraries and searches were used in order to assure complete coverage of the appropriate literature. Libraries used included medical libraries at the following institutions: The University of Connecticut Health Center, Farmington, Connecticut; Yale University Medical Library, New Haven, Connecticut; The Medical University of South Carolina Library, Charleston, South Carolina; The University of South Carolina Medical School Library and the Cooper Library, Columbia, South Carolina. The psychiatric library at The Institute of Living, Hartford, Connecticut was also used. Other libraries included the university libraries at The University of South Carolina-Coastal Carolina College, Conway, South Carolina; The University of South Carolina-Spartanburg, South Carolina; The University of South Carolina, Columbia, South Carolina; and Clemson University, Clemson, South Carolina.

The late Dr. Francis Braceland, a Director of the Institute of Living, allowed the author access to his personal files on the CMHC movement during her early research in the late 1970s. The files contained published works as well as unpublished drafts of Dr. Braceland's testimony to the United States Congress on behalf of the original CMHC legislation and early drafts of sections from Action for Mental Health.

ACTION FOR MENTAL HEALTH

Articles and books chosen for inclusion in this analysis were drawn from generally well regarded journals and widely distributed books. For the analysis of the conflict literature, the definition of acceptable sources of literature was widened a bit, but only to include sources in general distribution during the 1960s. Appropriate mainstream sources were identified through their common adoption by medical and psychiatric libraries, and by reputation as judged by this author and key informants. The decision whether to include works in the analysis was made on the basis of their relationship to the CMHC literature as a whole and their common availability. The sources used in the analysis were purposely chosen in this way in order to judge trends in the mainstream CMHC literature. The literatures of nursing and social work were not included since they were recognized as having their own unique histories and roles in the political economy of the movement.

Interviews were carried out with key informants who were knowledgeable about the CMHC movement. These interviews were used both to gather new data and to validate historical data and conclusions of the author. A series of interviews was carried out with Dr. Francis Braceland, one-time president of the American Psychiatric Association and active lobbyist for the CMHC movement during its early years. Dr. Louisa Howe, prominent clinical sociologist and CMHC theorist was also interviewed. Information about the middle years of the movement was gained from a daylong session with Dr. Michael Glen, founder and editor of *Radical Therapist*, a major anti-psychiatry journal of the late 1960s and early 1970s. The later years of the movement were explored during an interview with Dr. Gary Tishler, nationally prominent evaluation researcher and Study Director of the President's Commission on Mental Health during 1977-1978. Dr. Tishler was interviewed at Yale University.

METHOD OF ANALYSIS

The literature from the CMHC movement was chosen for inclusion in the study through analysis of key words in titles and in content. Articles and books were those which used the words "community mental health" in their titles or in their text. Appropriateness of other works was judged on the basis of their subject matter. For example, analyses of community participation and community development were judged to be salient issues for the movement, especially during the late 1960s, so articles on these topics were considered for inclusion.

As part of this research, ideal types of social theory were developed and applied to the CMHC literature. These types were based on classic ideal typical models. (See sources cited as appropriate in Chapters 2.) They were first applied to the analysis of the CMHC literature through use of key terms from each model such as system, subsystem, or consensus from the consensus model or class conflict, relations to the means of production, or cultural hegemony from the conflict model. Once the literature was sorted by this method into the general categories of consensus or conflict, a close reading of the piece was undertaken to judge its theoretical base. The fact that the ideal typical models were adapted from similar models, used in classic theory, provided a basis for judgements as to their importance.

The history of the CMHC movement constructed by the author was based on wide-ranging readings in CMHC history and validated through interviews with informants active in each period of the movement.

Models of state and market were drawn from classic works in political economy, specifically those of James O'Conner and Ernest Mandel. Although elaborations on these models have continued since their introduction, the author felt that their original formulations were adequate for the present purpose.

Overall validity of conclusions from the study were checked, whenever possible, through inter-source reliability, that is, through cross checking information in a number of written sources.

The analysis presented here is entirely the author's responsibility. Key informants did not read or approve the analysis or conclusions offered here.

Author Index

Subject Index

The Author

Dr. Sylvia Kenig has divided her professional efforts between traditional academe and applied sociology. A central theme of her work has been the integration of grand theory with sociological applications. She is an Assistant Professor of Sociology at the University of South Carolina–Coastal Carolina College. She has worked full-time as an independent consultant in evaluation research, specializing in the evaluation of health programs. Her publishing includes research on the community mental health centers movement, nursing in the South, and sexual harassment. Dr. Kenig received her B.A. from Goucher College and her M.A. and Ph.D. from the University of Connecticut.